the
Strength
of
Sensitivity

About the Author

Kyra Mesich, PsyD, earned a doctoral degree in clinical psychology from the Florida Institute of Technology. She also has received extensive training in the field of holistic health including flower essence therapy, yoga, meditation, mindfulness stress reduction, and Reiki energy healing.

Dr. Kyra has dedicated her career to supporting the holistic needs of sensitive people through individual sessions and workshops. She trains other health professionals to better recognize and help sensitive people, as well as how to incorporate holistic health practices into their work.

When not traveling for seminars and workshops, Dr. Kyra sees clients at her offices in Minneapolis and St. Paul, Minnesota. Visit her website www.drkyra.com.

Kyra Mesich, PsyD

the
Strength
of
Sensitivity

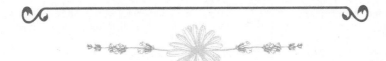

Understanding Empathy
for a Life of
Emotional Peace & Balance

Llewellyn Publications
Woodbury, Minnesota

FIRST EDITION
First Printing, 2016

Cover art: 62336634 © levgenila Lytvynovych/istockphoto.com
          62341150 © levgenila Lytvynovych/istockphoto.com
          62340542 © levgenila Lytvynovych/istockphoto.com
Cover design: Lisa Novak
Editing: Stephanie Finne
Interior part page art: 62336634 © levgenila Lytvynovych/istockphoto.com

Llewellyn Publications is a registered trademark of Llewellyn Worldwide Ltd.

Library of Congress Cataloging-in-Publication Data
Names: Mesich, Kyra, author.
Title: The strength of sensitivity : understanding empathy for a life of
   emotional peace & balance / by Kyra Mesich.
Description: First edition. | Woodbury, MN : Llewellyn Publications, [2016] |
   Includes bibliographical references and index.
Identifiers: LCCN 2015044364 (print) | LCCN 2016002333 (ebook) | ISBN
   9780738748498 | ISBN 9780738748733 ()
Subjects: LCSH: Sensitivity (Personality trait) | Empathy. | Mind and body.
Classification: LCC BF698.35.S47 M47 2016 (print) | LCC BF698.35.S47 (ebook)
   | DDC 158.2--dc23
LC record available at http://lccn.loc.gov/2015044364

Llewellyn Publications
A Division of Llewellyn Worldwide Ltd.
2143 Wooddale Drive
Woodbury, MN 55125-2989
www.llewellyn.com

Printed in the United States of America

Contents

Exercises & Meditations

Chapter 8

Appendix C

Disclaimer

The author of this book does not dispense medical advice or prescribe the use of any technique as a form of treatment for physical, emotional, or medical problems without the advice of a physician, either directly or indirectly. The material in this book is not intended as a substitute for trained medical or psychological advice. Readers are advised to consult their personal healthcare professionals regarding treatment. The intent of the author is only to offer information of a general nature to help you in your quest for emotional and spiritual well-being. The author and publisher assume no responsibility for your actions in the event you utilize any of the information in this book.

To the Sensitive Ones

Do not be ashamed of your sensitivity!
It has brought you many riches.

You see what others cannot see,
Feel what others are ashamed to feel.

You are more open, less numb.
You find it harder to turn a blind eye.

You have not closed your heart,
in spite of everything.

You are able to hold
the most intense highs
and the darkest lows
in your loving embrace.
(You know that neither define you.
Everything passes through.
You are a cosmic vessel.)

Celebrate your sensitivity!
It has kept you flexible and open.

You have remained close to wonder.
And awareness burns brightly in you.

Don't compare yourself with others.
Don't expect them to understand.

But teach them:
It's okay to feel, deeply.
It's okay to not know.
It's okay to play
on the raw edge of life.

Life may seem "harder" for you at times,
and often you are close to overwhelm.
But it's harder still
to repress your overwhelming gifts.

Sensitive ones,
Bring some gentleness into this weary world!
Shine on with courageous sensitivity!
You are the light bearers!
—Jeff Foster[1]

---

1. Jeff Foster, "To the Sensitive Ones," accessed Aug. 28, 2014, https://www.facebook
.com/LifeWithoutACentre.

Acknowledgments

I extend much gratitude to my editor, Angela Wix, for her unwavering patience and wise guidance. This book exists due to Angela's timing and input.

I acknowledge every single sensitive person who has come to my workshops, worked in private sessions, participated in studies, or has in any way taken the time to share their personal experience with me. Whether you know it or not, your contribution has brought shape to my work, and your willingness to learn about yourself will continue to help countless other sensitive people around the world.

There also is someone who would rather remain unnamed but who will recognize himself when I say his loving interest and curiosity has been the fundamental support to keep me on this path. Your love propels me to accomplish more than I think I can.

Introduction

This book took eighteen years to write.

Hello, I'm Dr. Kyra Mesich. I'm a holistic psychotherapist and proud to call myself a sensitive person. I wasn't always so proud, of course. My life began just like yours probably did—being misunderstood, picked on, and bullied, being told I was "too sensitive," wondering what the heck was wrong with me and why I was different. So in that way, I guess this book has really taken forty-five years to write.

These pages contain the sum of my journey thus far as a sensitive person. It will become pretty obvious to you as you read this book that a good part of my reason for being in this life has been to make sense, from a truly holistic perspective, of our sensitivity—not only to understand it, but also to turn sensitivity around and inside out into a positive, powerful way of being for us all.

I initially said it took me eighteen years to write this book, though, because that is when my professional psychology career took a turn. It very quickly veered in an unusual direction that I never could have predicted.

I've always been holistically minded, and I preferred integrating hypnosis and art into my psychotherapy sessions. I found conventional talk therapy sometimes missed the mark, and I felt it was inefficient. It didn't take me long at all as a young psychologist to fully realize that our human experience is like an iceberg.

More than 90 percent of an iceberg's volume and mass is under the water. There is only 10 percent that can be easily observed. And so it is with human beings. Taking into account our mind, emotions, spiritual energy, and intertwined physical symptoms, only 10 percent or so of who we really are can be easily accessed through conscious means such as talk therapy.

I felt that in a figurative sense, but before too long I was given a head-on, unforgettable example of some of that mysterious 90 percent.

A Life-Changing Experience

When I was a young psychologist, my first job after my internship was at a busy university counseling center. I worked with students and staff that had a myriad of issues and diagnoses. It was busy. It was interesting, and my coworkers were pretty great. All started out well.

But early one evening, I was suddenly hit out of the blue with a sickening depression. Over and over I thought, *I'm a failure. My life is hopeless.* I was shocked at myself for having such thoughts. I had struggled with depression plenty of times before in my life, but I'd never felt or thought those exact things before, and why would I at that moment? I didn't feel like a failure. I had just received my doctoral degree in psychology, and I was okay with my job and marriage. I didn't feel hopeless about anything at all.

Knowing that the thoughts were illogical certainly didn't stop them, though. The depression continued to spiral deeper through the night until I was overcome with sadness and hopelessness. I tried all the tricks I knew as a therapist to get my mind on a different track: exercise, distraction, journaling. Nothing was working. Finally, I decided to listen to some music. I put on my new Indigo Girls CD, but the sad theme of one of the songs penetrated to my heart like it never had before. It was a song of lost love, and it seemed to build upon my sadness until I was overcome with emotional pain. After scrawling in my journal about the unusual thoughts and intense pain of this depressive episode, wishing for it to stop, I fell asleep in tears.

The next morning, I woke up and it had passed. I was okay, and there was no reason for me not to go to work. My days began by greeting the office managers and retrieving my schedule. One of the receptionists said that a young man I had seen before named Dan had called to get an appointment right away because he said he had an emergency.

"Of course, I'll see him," I said. I wandered to my office wondering why Dan would have an emergency, as he wasn't the usual type. He suffered from mild depression and lack of direction in his life. He had been in counseling for several years, so he was very aware of his issues and usually would come in weekly whenever things were bothering him more. I soon would get my answer.

When Dan came in for his appointment, he plopped down on the blue couch, looking more defeated than ever. He said, "I had the worst depressive episode of my life last night, and it really scared me." As a dutiful young psychologist does, I pulled out my pen and notepad and said, "Oh, tell me about the events of last night."

Dan described how he had been romantically rebuffed by a young woman. He went out on what he thought was a date. It was not. He was embarrassed and felt rejected.

"When did that happen?" I asked.

"Early last evening," he replied. "So I hurried home and that's when I began sinking into a really deep depression."

Now remember that Dan had been in counseling for several years, so he actually was quite self-aware and knew the routine in a therapy session. He knew how to express himself. So he went on ...

"I started thinking about everything wrong in my life. Then negative thoughts repeated over and over in my mind, and I just couldn't stop them."

"What were those thoughts?" I inquired.

"I'm a failure. My life is hopeless."

The correlation was not lost on me. Dan had just described the time of the onset of my depressive episode the previous night and the exact thoughts that repeated over and over in my mind. From that moment forward, I'm sure Dan thought I was the most attentive therapist in the world as I began to search for anything that would make our simultaneous depressions a mere coincidence. But no differences were to be found.

Dan described how he tried to do the things he had learned in therapy to pull himself out of a depressive episode: distraction, calling a friend. He finally settled on listening to some music. He then thrust a crumpled up piece of paper toward me. "What's this?" I asked.

"It's a poem about my emotional pain. I wrote it last night," he replied.

"You've never done that before," I noted. "What prompted you to write this?"

Without a pause Dan replied, "Well, I was listening to my new Indigo Girls CD, and there was a song on there about lost love. I really resonated with the sadness of it, so I figured I would write about my pain, too."

"Ah, yes," I said, trying to maintain my appearance of steadfast impartiality. I glanced over the poem while my head was spinning.

I needed to close the session with Dan, so we did some cognitive reframing about what really happened with his female friend and how it didn't truly reflect upon him as a person nor relate to the possibilities for his life. Dan left the session feeling better.

I asked the secretaries to give me a few moments and closed my door. I felt dizzy to say the least. Dan had just perfectly described the painful depressive episode that had suddenly loomed over me the night before. There were way too many similarities for it to be coincidence: the time of onset, the thoughts, the quality of the depression. Then the song was like a cosmic joke—just in case I might be inclined to brush it all away as coincidence.

On one hand, it was a relief to have a valid cause for why I was suddenly overcome with such a powerful, unusual depression. It wasn't mine. But that realization—that I was experiencing someone else's emotions—was overwhelming and mystifying. At the time, I had no idea what to call this phenomena or what to do about it. So what was this event? To make a very long story short, it was an empathic experience. It was the first time I became aware of how empathic I was, and it helped me identify past and future empathic experiences. Thus began a long journey to understand just what empathic ability is and how it happens. Since there was so little information about it, I was determined to make sense of it. I especially wanted to figure out what types of people were empathic.

I eventually came to realize through hundreds of interviews with empaths, that empathic ability was always related to sensitivity. It was sensitive people who were the empaths. Since I myself was a highly sensitive person, I understood the relationship all too well.

Being empathic is being sensitive to emotional energy. It is vital to understand empathic ability in order to fully, holistically understand yourself as a sensitive person. In this book, you're going to learn about your sensitivity from that holistic perspective—body, mind, and spirit/ energy. Empathic ability falls under that spirit/energy heading.

The Strength of Sensitivity is a follow-up to a book I wrote in 2000 titled *The Sensitive Person's Survival Guide*. That book was, as the title implies, more about enduring the discomforts of being a sensitive, empathic person. In the fifteen years since I wrote the survival guide, I've learned a great deal about going beyond merely surviving, and instead learned to evolve my experience as a sensitive, empathic person. Empathic ability can be developed and used more comfortably. The way you experience your sensitivity can evolve, and its gifts and benefits can outweigh the overwhelm.

It is in that spirit that *The Strength of Sensitivity* was born. As sensitive people, our time has come to embrace who we are, carry ourselves proudly, and spread our influence to make the world a more peaceful, compassionate place.

It began with a crazy, uncomfortable experience that most people would have brushed away as a coincidence or "too weird." But that experience was pivotal to launch me into a deeper understanding and respect for sensitivity in all its manifestations.

I have deep respect for you, my dear reader, as a sensitive person. You embody much more strength than you know. You represent not only compassion and awareness, but also the connection all humans have to the realm of spirit/energy and to each other.

I want you to feel that respect for yourself. I also want you to know that the true strengths of your sensitivity are lying just below the surface of who you've been told you are as a sensitive person. You can redefine yourself and recalibrate your sensitivity, and you will then evolve in holistic, healing ways you have no idea of yet.

There is also one basic, yet very important, point that I want you to take away from *The Strength of Sensitivity* and that is: You are not alone! Sensitivity may feel isolating, but there are many, many of us out there.

How to Use This Book

This book is divided into three sections, and they build on each other in important ways. Each section has a distinctive theme to guide you along in your personal growth as a sensitive, perceptive person in this world.

Sorry to those who love to start with the last chapter first or flip open to the middle, but this book is designed to be read in the order of the chapters and sections. If you do skip ahead, I have tried to note when you may need to refer back to an important preceding idea. It's vital to challenge your own beliefs of who you are as a sensitive person, which you will learn in part 1, to be able to garner the most benefit from the ideas and tools in part 2.

Part 1 is about reframing and rethinking the notions we have accepted throughout life as people have told us who we are and what we should be as sensitive souls. Part 1 also introduces a truly holistic definition of sensitivity, with acknowledgment of our empathic, intuitive, and energetic awareness.

Part 2 moves on to sensitive recalibration. This section gives you motivation, tools, and ideas to actually reshape and transform how you experience your sensitivity. You aren't stuck and doomed to always be overwhelmed.

That progression leads to part 3, Sensitive (R)evolution! These are the most advanced ideas you'll find written anywhere to evolve your sensitivity from overwhelmed to overjoyed with all life has to offer.

Think of these three sections of the book as the parts of a flowering plant. So for a moment here, please visualize your favorite flower. Part 1, Sensitive Redefinition, is the roots that grow underground. It is the foundation from which everything else grows. The stem and leaves are part 2, Sensitive Recalibration, where chlorophyll transforms sunlight into energy that the plant uses to develop and grow. And the blooming flower is part 3, Sensitive (R)evolution, where the plant suddenly becomes something entirely different and distinctly beautiful. I've also included a lot of resources for you in the back of this book, including other writings that will elaborate on the concepts in these chapters.

This book touches on many different aspects of being a sensitive, perceptive person from a truly holistic perspective of body, mind, and spirit. Throughout the book you will be challenged to let go of all the stereotypes and limitations you learned to accept from others and subsequently have inflicted upon yourself. I hope you will keep this book on hand and refer back to it for years to come as you evolve, grow, and learn to appreciate and enjoy the strength of your sensitivity.

Part I

Sensitive
Redefinition

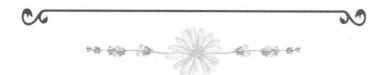

CHAPTER 1

Highly Sensitive vs. Highly Perceptive

Let's begin right away by acknowledging that sensitive people have gotten a horrible rap for centuries. I'm sure I don't need to tell you how sensitive people have been maligned, bullied, and outright abused. We live in a business-oriented and aggressive culture here in the United States. Therefore, the finer attributes of sensitivity have been trampled upon in favor of competition, loudness, and a numbing of the senses.

That's how it has been historically, anyway. But we are on the precipice of change. People in general are becoming more compassionate of their fellow humans (and animals), more inclined to work together for common goals, and more aware of their personal impact upon the earth and upon others.

That said, I know all too well that there are still individuals and groups out there who represent *in*sensitivity in all its forms. It's one step forward and two steps back sometimes. Yet, that is the very reason I've written this book. It's now time for sensitive people to make a stand. Our attributes of sensitivity are the very things that will save humanity in the long run. But before I get too high and mighty about the importance of sensitive people, please allow me to introduce you to a new perspective and a new way for you to think about your sensitivity.

I describe sensitive people as those of us who are very perceptive and aware of even subtle influences. We feel emotions deeply; experience strong reactions, both physical and emotional; and generally experience the world with more *impact* than less-sensitive people.

There are some common misunderstandings about what sensitivity is. Sensitivity is often confused with shyness and with introversion. These are separate concepts, though. Sensitivity is indicative of the way a person perceives and reacts to physical and emotional stimuli. Sensitive people are able to perceive even subtle stimuli and often experience very strong physiological reactions. This physiological tendency to be perceptive and responsive defines a person as sensitive. That sensitive person may or may not be shy and may even be an extrovert.

Shyness is the tendency to feel awkward, self-conscious, or tense during social encounters, especially with unfamiliar people. A sensitive person may be shy or may be quite comfortable around new people. The biggest confusion is with introversion vs. extroversion. Some people assume that all sensitive people are introverts, but this is not so.

Whether someone is an introvert or an extrovert has to do with how they utilize their energy when around other people. For example, at a party, the extroverts are the ones who will stay late chatting until all hours because they never seem to get tired. In fact, extroverts become more and more energized as they interact with people. Introverts, on the other hand, are those who will have fun for a while and then want to leave because they become tired. Introverts utilize their own energy as the fuel for social situations, so eventually the introvert's energy becomes depleted and it's time to go home.

I have met many sensitive extroverts at my workshops. So, yes, a person may be a shy, sensitive introvert, but another sensitive person may be an unabashed extrovert ... or any combination thereof. I myself am sensitive and an introvert, but I'm not in the slightest bit shy. They are all separate aspects of our being that sometimes intermingle. I hope that clarifies what sensitivity is not. Now let's get back to what sensitivity is.

I'll present two different lists of the traits of sensitivity. First, I'll give you the old, familiar list, which is a bit more frustration and symptom oriented. Then we'll move on to the new list, which turns 180 degrees from how we normally think of ourselves as sensitive people.

Traits of Sensitivity: The Old List

The following is the classic list of the traits of sensitivity. Admittedly, it was the list I used in my first book fifteen years ago.

1. Sensitive people feel emotions often and deeply. They feel as if they "wear their emotions on their sleeves."

2. They are keenly aware of the emotions of people around them.

3. Sensitive people are easily hurt or upset. An insult or unkind remark will affect them deeply.

4. In a similar vein, sensitive people strive to avoid conflicts. They dread arguments and other types of confrontations because the negativity affects them so much.

5. Sensitive people are not able to shake off emotions easily. Once they are saddened or upset by something, they cannot just switch gears and forget it.

6. Sensitive people are greatly affected by emotions they witness. They feel deeply for others' suffering. Many sensitive people avoid sad movies, violent images, or watching the news because they cannot bear the weighty emotions that would drive to their core and stick with them afterward.

7. Sensitive people are prone to suffer from recurrent depression or anxiety.

8. On the positive side, sensitive people are also keenly aware of and affected by positivity and beauty in art, music, and nature. They are the world's greatest artists and art appreciators.

9. Related to number eight, sensitive people are often creative. Even if they are not artists, they are generally able to "think outside the box."

10. Sensitive people are prone to stimulus overload and overwhelm. That is, they can't stand large crowds, loud noise, or hectic environments. They feel depleted by too much stimuli.

11. Similarly, sensitive people often startle easily and have a nervous system that is easily frazzled.

12. Sensitive people are empathic and know what needs to be done to make other people comfortable or feel better.

13. Sensitive people are naturally intuitive and do best when they follow their gut instincts.

14. Sensitive people are born that way. They were sensitive children. There are a couple different responses kids have to their sensitivity. One type of sensitive child is the stereotypical kid who gets picked on by bullies and is a well-behaved, quiet student because he or she cannot stand the thought of getting into trouble. The other type of sensitive child more often experiences the stimulus overload mentioned above. These children are thus overstimulated much of the time and have difficulty focusing, which causes them problems in school and in relationships.

Sensitive people typically experience all or nearly all of the above situations in their lives. This list isn't finished, though, until I mention this underlying, universal attitude:

One of the sure signs of a truly sensitive person is that he or she feels animosity toward his or her sensitive nature. Most sensitive people whole-heartedly wish they were tougher and more thick-skinned. They feel like (and have been told) their sensitivity is a weakness. They wish things didn't bother them so much. They wish their emotions weren't so obvious to other people. They wish they could let things go and not worry so much. They aren't comfortable with their sensitivity, and they wish they could do something to get rid of it (or at least get rid of the uncomfortable aspects of it). They are tired of feeling overwhelmed.

Obviously, much of this self-dissatisfaction is not inherent to being a sensitive person. It is a product of the family and the society in which we live.

Now, there are definitely some positive qualities in this list: keen awareness, creativity, emotional discernment, and intuitive gifts. But this old way of conceptualizing sensitivity centers on the discomfort and overwhelm we experience as sensitive people. Thus, it leaves many sensitive people feeling that there is nothing useful nor good about their sensitive nature. I have had plenty of sensitive people come to my workshops and say, "Why am I this way? Why am I different? There is nothing positive nor helpful about the way I am."

Traits of Sensitivity: The New List

In response to this, please join me in a shift of perspective to reiterate and rephrase the traits of sensitivity. All of these have been demonstrated in research and observation. This is my *new* list of the traits of sensitivity:

1. Acute, sharp sensory processing
2. Greater brain activity in response to stimuli
3. Powerful emotions
4. Quick reactions by our nervous systems
5. Strong autonomic responses in our body (digestive, heart, and other organ responses)
6. Empathic, conscientious, and compassionate
7. Creative with an appreciation for art and beauty
8. Very perceptive with awareness of energies from others and the environment
9. Intuitive with good gut instincts
10. Love of nature

The old list of attributes is an inventory of experiences that sensitive people easily relate to, and that is because it focuses more on the struggles and discomfort we face. In that way, the old list helps a sensitive person feel not so alone with their overwhelmed senses. You can feel reassured that you are not the only one. There are a lot of us sensitive people out there feeling the same things you do.

But please reread my second list and notice that exactly the same experiences are there, just rephrased from a different viewpoint. There is absolutely nothing in the new list that indicates weakness or that anything is wrong with us at all as sensitive people. Much to the contrary, actually. Review the adjectives I've used in the new list: *acute, powerful, greater, quick, strong, perceptive, conscientious, creative, intuitive*, and *love*. These are all great and powerful strengths!

I want you to begin to shift your own beliefs about your sensitivity. We are not by any means weak or defective. We are, in fact, more effective, more highly responsive, and our senses and bodily systems are more aware and perceptive.

· ·
Sensitivity Free Association Writing Exercise

We've spent a good amount of time talking about sensitivity in terms of generalities, but now I'd like you to turn your attention to your own life and consider your own feelings about your sensitivity.

For this exercise, write the word "Sensitivity" in big letters across the top of a piece of paper. Go ahead and do that now. Under the heading, write down every association that occurs to you when you think of sensitivity. This is brainstorming free association. Don't censor yourself and don't overthink it. Write down every word, thought, feeling, or memory that comes up for you when you think of the word. Write for as long as the train of thought continues. One idea may lead to another, and that's fine.

Once you've completed the free association list, go back and look over what you wrote. Divide out your list by what associations seem positive, which are negative, and maybe some will be neutral. The point of this exercise is for you to be honest with yourself and aware of how you really feel about being a sensitive person.

· ·

I hope you have some positive associations in your list. We all have mixed feelings about being sensitive. But for many of us "sensitive" is a loaded word. It's a term that has effectively been ruined by the connotations of our society. The word "sensitive," which should only mean "having acute senses," has been burdened by our society to immediately mean "too sensitive" and conjure up additional notions like weak, sissy, crybaby, easy target, etc. Those associations are wrong. They are unfortunate, but it's the way it has been. So although you may be able to agree with me intellectually that sensitivity has many positive attributes and should be appreciated, the old emotionally laden associations may linger.

If this is the case for you, for the remainder of this book, I invite you to no longer describe yourself as highly sensitive. Instead, I want you to think of yourself as *highly perceptive*.

We aren't giving up on the word "sensitive" by any means. I'll still use it throughout this book, but I want to give you an opportunity to take a break from defining yourself with a word that has been tainted with old negative overtones. *Highly Perceptive* is a neutral term that gives you a chance to think about your traits of sensitivity in an unbiased way. You can always go back to describing yourself as sensitive later if you wish.

This discussion demonstrates how words can be touchy things that often incite emotions and sometimes downright defensiveness. "Sensitive" is one of those particularly tricky words. It has associations that incite reactions in both directions. There may be people who will take offense to my use of the term "less sensitive." They'll say, "Hey! I'm not insensitive!" and feel like I am saying they are "lesser" in comparison to those of us who are more sensitive. In general, no one wants to be called too sensitive or not sensitive enough. In this book, there is no judgment toward either side. We all fall somewhere on the continuum, and we are all of value.

Reframing Old Negative
Overtones and Discomfort

In my workshops, I often receive questions in response to my new list of positively inclined sensitive descriptors. The first question is usually, "So, Dr. Kyra, if we're just more perceptive, intuitive, and aware, then why have we been bullied and put down for so long?"

That's a fair question. I, of course, don't know the complete answer, but much of it lies in what I'll be discussing in future chapters about the body-mind-spirit links of sensitivity. Suffice it for now to say that we, as sensitive people, make less-aware people very uncomfortable. We notice what they don't want to notice. We react to the dangerous things they don't want to stop doing or making. We crave peace and cooperation, while they insist upon competition and an "every man for himself" mentality.

To put it bluntly, we are in the way. We don't go along with the conventional status quo. Whether we mean to or not, our sensitivity draws attention to the faults, the abuses, and the negativity of our society's (and our family's) choices. To put it more simply, our sensitive reactions (physical, emotional, and energetic) illuminate what is unbalanced and what isn't working ... for *everyone*, not just for our sensitive selves. And this is the very reason we need to claim our collective strength as sensitive people and recognize our importance in the scheme of things.

Now, of course, I'm not implying we should set up an adversarial relationship with those who are not as highly sensitive. It doesn't help anyone for us to be judgmental, even if we feel we have been judged in the past. Instead, as sensitive people, our skill is our ability to work toward acceptance and inclusivity. The key is for us to value our sensitivity enough that we expect that acceptance and cooperation in return, then we can all be equals and work to solve some of those imbalances together.

Other questions that often follow are: "If I'm made up of highly perceptive strengths, then why am I uncomfortable so much of the time? Why does it hurt to be me?"

There are ways to greatly reduce the discomforts related to being sensitive. To start, we need to reframe how we think about and refer to the discomfort that we are feeling.

First of all, consider for a moment the truth of the matter. Our environment and surroundings are often unnecessarily intense, loud, unhealthy, and unbalanced. We are not responding to nothing. If we are feeling bombarded or uncomfortable, then our body is generally reacting to a bona fide unhealthy stimulus. Doesn't it make sense that when we're being exposed to a stimulus such as noxious chemicals, a very stressful work environment, a cacophony of discordant noises, or a rude, nasty person, that we *should* experience a response that indicates how unhealthy or unbalanced the situation is?

Although negative, unhealthy stimuli might be prevalent, the less-sensitive person doesn't feel the impetus to make any changes. For example, exposure to noxious chemicals on the job might be giving a less-sensitive person headaches or brain fog, but it doesn't occur to him to find the danger and eliminate it. Obviously, that won't be good for him at all in the long run, and he may even become incapacitated in a short amount of exposure time. All because he didn't quickly notice the discomfort and take action to change the situation.

Follow what I'm saying? The discomfort we feel as sensitive people can often be reframed as our body's or our psyche's way of telling us to reduce or eliminate an unhealthy, unbalanced situation.

We've all heard it numerous times: "You're being *too* sensitive." That's an unhelpful commentary that doesn't have anything to do with what we are experiencing within. Our sensitive, perceptive reactions, on the other hand, don't care at all about how society would have us react to a stimulus. Our body is neutral, and it simply is attempting to communicate what we need to know to protect ourselves and to live healthier and longer.

You've likely been given messages your whole life that you are "too sensitive" with add-ons such as "You're making a big deal out of nothing."

Most of us sensitive people have had to endure messages from various sources throughout our entire lives that we were too touchy, weak, and weird; we didn't fit in; and that something was wrong with us because we were sensitive. Therefore, dear perceptive reader, if you are anything like the rest of us, you have accepted those unkind messages as your own beliefs about who you are. Those judgments from others become a core part of our identity. Here are some examples of the beliefs sensitive people often have about themselves:

- I am too sensitive.
- I can't cope.
- I am odd, no one understands me.
- I get picked on and bullied.
- I care too much.

This is a rough self-image to carry around through life, and it was formed by other people's unhelpful comments and unhealthy reactions to us. When we're young, we readily go into that "box" that other people pigeonhole us into. Unfortunately, this "contaminated" self-image can be a very stubborn thing to change, even once you begin to realize it isn't true. I've witnessed the resistance in client after client after client.

But, no worries, we are just getting started. Trust me, by the end of this book I will have given you evidence that all those blaming, judgmental, unhelpful labels you may have grown up with were simply wrong.

The Strength of Sensitivity

Highly perceptive, sensitive people may be in the minority, but sensitivity is not indicative of weakness. It is strength of consciousness, awareness, and perception, and that can leave the less-sensitive person a little baffled, if not downright uncomfortable.

Another opinion I'd like you to modify about your sensitivity is that you are odd or strange. Sensitivity is actually not as rare as you might think. According to Dr. Elaine Aron, author of *The Highly Sen-*

sitive Person, we are about 20 percent of the population.[2] Twenty percent is a minority, yes, but it's a pretty large one, and definitely significant enough to make an impact on the world.

I know all too well that our self-perception is not easily swayed, and it may be hard to accept the positives of that second list about the strengths of sensitivity. So let's talk about some of those strengths a little more and break down the list.

1. Acute, sharp sensory processing

This one shouldn't be too hard for you to resonate with. As sensitive people, we often find ourselves as the ones who smell the odd odor others don't notice, hear the high-pitched sound others are deaf to, have to wear sunglasses when others don't seem to mind the bright sunlight, can't stand the itchy tags in our new clothing, and taste the nuances of the recipe (for better or worse). Our five senses, quite frankly, work better and are more perceptive than those of less-sensitive people.

Dr. Aron and her husband and colleagues at Stony Brook University coined the term "sensory processing sensitivity." This is a more scientific way of saying that a sensitive person's five physical senses of sight, hearing, smell, touch, and taste are more acute and effective than the average person's.[3]

And I'll add that we gain advantages from our superior senses, which include more than just our five senses. I include empathic ability and intuition as well.

2. Greater brain activity in response to stimuli

It's time to cite another study from Dr. Aron and colleagues. In this study, the participants' brain activity was monitored by functional magnetic resonance imaging while they viewed a series of photos of

2. Elaine Aron, "Is this You?," accessed Jan. 2015, http://hsperson.com.

3. Elaine Aron, Arthur Aron, and Jadzia Jagiellowicz, "Sensory Processing Sensitivity: A Review in the Light of the Evolution of Biological Responsivity," *Personality and Social Psychology Review* Vol. 16, No. 3 (2012): 262–282.

people exhibiting varied emotions.[4] The participants were divided into the categories of highly sensitive or not sensitive. Findings: The sensitive participants had much greater blood flow in their brains, indicating higher brain activity. Additional imaging studies have also been done showing similar results with more neutral cognitive stimuli.[5]

This leads to a change in thought about exactly what sensitivity is. How often have we been dismissed with "Oh, you're just being too sensitive," as if our sensitive reactions were just ethereal nothingness that we somehow magically imagined or made up. To the contrary, this MRI study resulted in concrete evidence that sensitivity and our powerful reactions to stimuli are physiological, hard-wired responses of our body. We're sensitive because our entire physiology—our brain, our nervous system, our cellular structure—is indeed more reactive, responsive, and perhaps we could even say more powerful. We're not making it up, folks.

3. Powerful emotions

This is another trait that should have a familiar ring to it. As sensitive people, we often feel and express strong emotions in response to an event, a movie, a news story, or even a passing comment from someone.

This tendency for powerful emotions was also evidenced in the MRI study I referenced above. Sensitive participants had the greatest brain activity when they viewed photos of their own partner as happy. I use this example to explain why I think powerful emotions are a strength of character. We are able to experience positive emotions in a fantastically intense way.

I know what you're thinking though, "Excuse me, Dr. Kyra, but my powerful emotions are not a strength when I have to hide crying at

4. Bianca Acevedo, Elaine Aron, Arthur Aron, Matthew-Donald Sangster, Nancy Collins, and Lucy Brown, "The Highly Sensitive Brain: An fMRI Study of Sensory Processing Sensitivity and Response to Others' Emotions," *Brain and Behavior* Vol. 4, No. 4 (2014): 580–594.

5. Jadzia Jagiellowicz, Xiaomeng Xu, Arthur Aron, Elaine Aron, Guikang Cao, Tingyong Feng, and XuchuWeng, "The Trait of Sensory Processing Sensitivity and Neural Responses to Changes in Visual Scenes," *Social Cognitive and Affective Neuroscience* Vol. 6, No. 1 (2011): 38–47.

work or when a stupid commercial brings me to tears." We'll get more into that type of emotional management, but stick with me for the moment. We feel *all* emotions deeply. Therefore, we feel positive emotions with more intensity as well, and I consider that a rewarding way to live.

Lest you think that emotions really aren't useful or good for anything, there are researchers who would disagree. An interesting article titled "The Emotions That Make Us More Creative"[6] cites several researchers' work to understand the relationships among emotions, attention, focus, and creativity.

In summary, researchers found that very strong emotions, both positive and negative, led to something they called "motivational intensity," the internal force to create and accomplish. This was seen as a good thing in both artistic and work environments. Researchers also found that "affective engagement"—the extent to which people are open to the full breadth and depth of their emotions—was the best predictor of artistic creativity.

So even from what may seem like a disengaged scientific perspective, emotions are seen as fuel, necessary for increased focus and motivation and allowing for greater creativity. Intense feelings aren't all bad. They make us who we are.

But, yes, we will address how to lessen the intensity of the painful, negative emotions that may be plaguing you as a sensitive person in part 2 of this book.

The Subtler Aspects of Sensitivity

I imagine you're beginning to get the point now about the positive traits in my new strengths of sensitivity list, so I don't need to overstate my case by explicitly identifying the wonderfulness of all ten items. Numbers 1, 2, and 3 that we just discussed are concepts that are easy to understand: the keen sensitivity of our five senses, our body's physiological reactions, and our sensitive emotions. These are the

---

6. Barry Scott Kaufman, "The Emotions That Make Us More Creative," accessed Aug. 15, 2015, https://hbr.org/2015/08/the-emotions-that-make-us-more-creative.

"body" and "mind" pieces of the body-mind-spirit triad. There are two more, though, that I want to highlight right now because they are essentially the core theme of this book:

8. Very perceptive with awareness of energies from others and the environment
9. Intuitive with good gut instincts

But, uh oh, numbers 8 and 9 have now slipped into that mystical third segment, "spirit," which we could also call "energy," "etheric," "metaphysical," or "quantum." Whichever term you want to use, with numbers 8 and 9 we've now dared to step outside mainstream prejudice into what I consider to be the true domain of sensitive people.

And what is this domain? I call it the "*subtleties*" of life experience. As sensitive people, we are very aware of even the most subtle influences around us. So for now, let's just use the catch-all term "energy." Sensitive people can perceive and sense the impact of the energy that surrounds us in all its forms.

The remainder of this book will discuss just that in much more depth. We'll address the body, mind, and spirit aspects of sensitivity, but especially the less-understood spirit/energetics of sensitivity.

Since good work, such as that of Dr. Elaine Aron, has already been put forth in support of sensitive people, what I aim to do in this book is uncover the important topics that I feel have been overlooked thus far. I am an alternative-minded, holistic health practitioner. Right now, I'm not affiliated with a university or any other institution that would force my writing to be more mainstream, so I can write about *all* aspects of sensitivity, including the metaphysical.

In fact, my work over the past fifteen years has proven to me that acknowledgment of the energetic, metaphysical, quantum components of sensitivity is the only thing that truly allows us to manage and reduce the discomfort associated with our sensitivity. I'll say that one more time a little more succinctly. We have no means to reduce the pain and frustrations of being sensitive, *unless* we also include the energetic, subtle realms of ourselves and our world into the equation. When we do, we have the means for much greater understanding of ourselves and our sensitive reactions.

Knowing that 20 percent of the population is highly sensitive is great. Then we know we are not alone. Being aware of some tips for how to manage the physical sensory overload we sometimes experience is also helpful. But it is vital that we sensitive souls embrace a holistic view of ourselves as sensitive creatures. It's not until we embrace body, mind, *and* the energetic aspects of sensitivity, that we have any means to even begin to understand who we really are and *what* it really is that we are responding to. A holistic, energetic viewpoint results in the tools and methods to actually *change* our experience of our sensitivity. That is, we can make it more comfortable and useful to us. With the third, quantum, part of our sensitivity uncovered, we can change and evolve our sensitivity in more effective ways than we ever thought possible.

So turn the page, and we'll plunge right in to the energetic side of our sensitivity.

CHAPTER 2

Introduction to Energetic & Empathic Sensitivity

Counter to conventional standards, I'm going against the traditional order of body, mind, and spirit. Notice how spirit is always mentioned last? In this book, spirit/energy, aka the metaphysical aspect of your being (whatever term you want to use), is *first*! How's that for a mini-rebellion?

I'm doing this because as sensitive people we need to understand that we are more aware of *everything* and especially that which is energetic. For someone who is less sensitive, it's easy for him or her to discount the ethereal and say, "I'll believe it when I see it," even though that is an incredibly illogical statement.

Let's start with the obvious invisible energies we live amongst every day. We are continually surrounded by energies that we cannot see: radiation; signals from cell phone towers; microwaves; electromagnetic frequencies from televisions, computers, high power lines, and on and on. And that's not even to mention the molecularly sized bacteria and viruses that affect our health in sometimes extreme ways. We're being impacted at all times by an environment teeming with invisible energies we cannot see. What makes the sensitive person different in our electromagnetic environment? We are the ones who are often able to sense and feel the effects this energy has on our bodies. Sometimes it is not so subtle to us.

Is that a weakness? Of course not! Isn't it preferable to be aware and able to sense how these invisible energies may be affecting us? That way we can make choices as necessary for our health and well-being.

Now let's take this discussion of invisible energies one logical step further. We, human beings, are made of skin, salt water, and electrical charges. We are electrical and energetic in nature. It is no secret that electrical charges pulsate throughout our bodies. EEGs measure electrical activity in the neurons of the brain. EKGs measure electrical activity in the heart. These electrical measurements are used by medical practitioners every single day. Yet, in our day-to-day lives we somehow forget that we have these energetic impulses coursing through our bodies constantly. In science classes, we learn that neurons communicate by sending electrical signals throughout the body. Every single cell, every single nerve in our body communicates through an electrochemical language. We are composed of electrical and energetic frequencies.

In addition to physical movement, every thought and every feeling generates a complex electrical current as neurons fire.[7] This has been discussed in works such as *The Body Electric* by Robert Becker, MD.

Even more scientists than you might think admit to the mysterious, entangled energetic field that is our mental and emotional experience. A good example is the book *Everything You Need to Know to Feel Go(o)d* by Candace Pert, PhD. Dr. Pert was Chief of Brain Biochemistry at the National Institutes of Health. She was a highly regarded scientist, a leader in her field, and obviously, a sensitive person. She took the time in her research of brain biochemistry to notice and ponder how it related to the nuances and depth of human experience.

Dr. Pert said, "We're not just little hunks of meat. We're vibrating like a tuning fork—we send out a vibration to other people. We broad-

---

7. Elizabeth Dougherty, "What Are Thoughts Made Of?", accessed March 1, 2015, http://engineering.mit.edu/ask/what-are-thoughts-made.

cast and receive." She also clarified, "Mainstream science doesn't explain how one person's emotions can affect another person and the larger world. People still think about this as chemistry … Of course it is chemistry, but it's also physics and vibrations."[8]

With acknowledgment of our electrical field and human-generated energetic vibrations, we have moved beyond the mechanistic and superficial. We now enter the realm of quantum physics. We emit energy. We vibrate. We are just barely beginning to scientifically understand this energetic part of who we are, but as sensitive people, we have felt it all along. Whether we are aware of it or not, we are emitters and receptors of emotional energy, and that fact turns our view to the misunderstood concept of empathic ability.

Empathic Sensitivity

In the introduction, you read my story of the intense empathic experience that forced me to establish an entirely new understanding of emotions and sensitivity. Not everyone has such clear and profound empathic experiences, of course. There are many ways empathic ability is expressed. First, let me lay out a thorough definition of empathic ability. This is a concept that we simply don't talk about in our culture, so it's time to change that. We'll take this in stages.

We'll start first with the common concept of empathy. The Merriam-Webster dictionary definition of empathy is "the action of understanding, being aware of, being sensitive to, and vicariously experiencing the feelings, thoughts, and experience of another of either the past or present without having the feelings, thoughts, and experience fully communicated in an objectively explicit manner."[9] Sensitive people find themselves experiencing a great deal of empathy for the plights of their fellow humans and animals.

---

8. Joshua Freedman, "The Physics of Emotion: Candace Pert on Feeling Go(o)d," accessed July 5, 2015, http://www.6seconds.org/2007/01/26/the-physics-of-emotion-candace-pert-on-feeling-good.

9. Merriam-Webster dictionary, "Empathy," accessed June 30, 2015, http://www.merriam-webster.com/dictionary/empathy.

We experience sympathy, too, but empathy is quite different from sympathy. Sympathy is the feeling that you care about and are sorry about someone else's trouble, grief, or misfortune. As in, "Hey, buddy, whoa, that must have been rough. Let's go out for a beer, and you'll feel better." Empathy on the other hand is, "Oh no, buddy, how awful! I know exactly how you feel. Please let me know if there is any way I can help you. I'm here with you." There is distance with sympathy. "I feel bad that you're in pain. I hope you get over it soon." With empathy there is very little, if any, separateness. "I feel your pain."

In this book, the terms *empathy*, *empathic*, *empathetic*, *empathic ability*, and a couple others all refer to this same concept of literally sharing another person's emotional experience.

So, ponder this with me ... our culture is willing to define empathy up to this point, "vicariously experiencing the feelings of another, even without the feeling having been fully communicated." Stated more simply, the ability to experience someone else's feelings, whether she told you about them or not.

Then the definition of empathy stops there. It just stops. No further explanation is pondered nor even wanted by the general public. But as a sensitive, empathic person, we wonder *why*? Why do I cry and feel this other person's pain? Why do I feel so intensely that it hurts my insides when many people are affected by a tragedy? Why do I seem to understand other people's emotions even better than they themselves do? How on earth does this sharing and vicarious emotional experience happen? Sensitive people often end this line of thought with the question, "And how do I change it so I don't hurt so much?" That is the big question we'll be addressing soon, and, believe it or not, there actually is an answer. Dr. Pert alluded to it in her quotes earlier in this chapter. People still think of emotions as purely chemistry. As Dr. Pert said, "Of course it is chemistry, but it's also physics and vibrations." In other words, it is *energy*.

So here is my new energetic definition of empathy: "Empathic awareness is the purest form of emotional communication. Some call it the most advanced of all communication skills. It is the straight processing of emotional energy, unimpeded by intellectual filters.

Neither passage of time, words, nor physical observation are required with empathic communication."

Empathic communication can happen instantaneously, across any distance. It is quantum, and the experience can range from a subtle, barely discernible feeling to a profound emotional or physical symptom.

Empathic ability is a reminder that we are all connected by an invisible ether of emotional current that intermingles with our own biofrequencies. I am using the term "emotional" in this discussion for simplicity. Keep in mind that we are body, mind, and spirit all entangled. There is no hard boundary between thoughts, emotions, physical symptoms, etc. Any of these can and are communicated empathically. When there is any kind of feeling component to the energy, then your empathic awareness can perceive that energetic current of emotional vibration.

Here are examples of energetic/empathic sensitivity and how it might manifest in your life.

1. Direct transfer of emotional energy from another person or group
2. Awareness of the emotional energetic vibration of an environment or a place
3. Emotional/mental overwhelm in a crowded, loud, or chaotic situation
4. Accurate "gut feelings" about another's character or trustworthiness
5. Deep awareness of the emotional energy of domestic and/or wild animals
6. Feeling stuck with old emotions, particularly after an argument or a negative interaction
7. Feeling others' physical discomfort or symptoms
8. A natural ability to know how to make others feel comfortable
9. Others are drawn to you for advice and may "dump" their worries on you or otherwise take advantage of your kindness

10. Thinking or problem solving in a creative, outside the box, intuitive way

11. Deep connection with the meaning of art and a desire to use it for your own emotional expression. This also applies to the beauty of nature.

12. Inexplicable depression or anxiety that is unrelated to your life circumstances

Let's take a look at each of these in more detail.

Empathic Sensitivity #1
Direct transfer of emotional energy from another person or group

This is the image most people come up with when conceptualizing an empathic person, like Counselor Deanna Troi on *Star Trek: The Next Generation*. The empath has useful skills but can sometimes be overwhelmed by the intensity of experiencing another's energy so directly.

An example of this type of empathic experience would be feeling off or depressed for no apparent reason, and then having a friend call you with sad news that happened to her. The grief is communicated empathically, in a quantum manner, well in advance of the physical delivery of the message.

Empathic Sensitivity #2
Awareness of the emotional energetic vibration of an environment or a place

I think all sensitive people have had at least one or two experiences in their lives of feeling the energy of a place. That can be a fantastic feeling of being overcome with the peacefulness and powerful energy of a beautiful natural place such as a forest or a beach. It also can be experienced as an uncomfortable "I can't stay here" feeling. Usually that uneasy feeling means that some people left residual energy in that place. Depending upon the location, it could be sadness, anger, fear, grief, or even something like chaotic energy from drug use.

It doesn't matter that we don't understand *how* these vibrations linger. We aren't at that point in our ability to understand and measure quantum emotional energy. But the fact remains that it does happen, and sensitive people can empathically feel that energetic climate, no matter how subtle it might be.

Empathic Sensitivity #3
Emotional/mental overwhelm in a crowded, loud, or chaotic situation

Of course, there are some purely physiological reasons for this type of overwhelm in overstimulating situations. As I discussed in chapter 1, sensitive people have highly active and responsive nervous systems, which can lead to feeling depleted from too much stimuli. But, by now you know my mantra for this book—body, mind, and energy are inextricably intertwined. Where there is a physical sensation, there is also an energetic component.

Remember what Dr. Pert said, we aren't just made of chemicals. We are the embodiment of physics and vibrations. When we are in a very crowded or chaotic environment, there is a heck of a lot of quantum vibration going on. It makes sense that as sensitive people, we are aware of all of it. It would be one thing if we were in a crowded environment of healthy, happy, grounded, lighthearted people having a fun time. We would be feeling pretty good, no matter how big the crowd.

As a matter of fact, someone recently told me a story that illustrated just this point. He was very nervous to be going to a huge music concert. He normally felt very uncomfortable and depleted from crowded situations, and this concert was going to have an attendance of seventy thousand people! He thought it would be impossible to enjoy himself, but it was an important event for his wife, so he agreed to go along.

His report: He was absolutely shocked that at this particular concert of a classic band the mood of the crowd was very positive overall. He said that people were polite and obviously having a lot of fun.

Most everyone appeared very happy to be there. So as a sensitive person, not only was he okay, but he began to feel an immense uplifting feeling. It turned out to be an incredible, positive wave of energy that he was able to fully sense and ride for the entire night.

What a fabulous experience to be empathic in a happy world! But, unfortunately, most crowds contain a mix. Some people are peaceful and contented, but there will most always be a varying percentage of people who are angry, upset, possibly way too inebriated, or otherwise unbalanced, depending on the occasion.

So, again, let's consider. Is it a weakness to perceive the huge variety of energies in a crowded place? No, it's simply feeling the complex truth of the environment. It allows us to perhaps shift or move within the environment to find the people who are emitting the most balanced energy.

But, yes, I know that sometimes we have to be in those unhealthy, crowded, crazy situations. And sometimes we want to be able to deal with such a place even when we know it's going to be a mixed bag.

Empathic Sensitivity #4
Accurate "gut feelings" about another's character or trustworthiness

There is a blurred line between "empathic ability" and "intuition." Sometimes I even find myself using the terms interchangeably as I try to explain to someone why I made a certain choice. "Because my intuition told me to" is often my default answer. Empathic, gut feelings, intuitive hunches—they all are an expression of the metaphysical, energetic aspect of our being. We can't explain *how* we know or feel something. We just *do*, and most of us learn the hard way that circumstances don't work out so well when we ignore our gut feelings.

The fact is that most sensitive people have a really strong, highly accurate intuitive empathic meter that gives us a feeling about each person we encounter. It can be, "Hey, I connect with this person easily!" It may be neutral. Or, "Er, I don't know about that guy." As sensitive people, upon spending a little time with someone, we often have a pretty clear twinge of energy within us that indicates how our dealings with that person will turn out. Sometimes it is a very subtle feeling. A lot of times we ignore gut feelings or intellectualize them away. But it's there, and the more we pay attention to it, the easier our dealings with people become.

I sometimes hear the following: "Dr. Kyra, people often turn out different than I expect and disappoint me." My response? Either your brain or your old emotional patterns (or both) are overriding your empathic awareness and intuition. Please look back at my sentence in the previous paragraph: *A lot of times we ignore gut feelings or intellectualize them away*. If people often turn out to have a different character than you expected, then your brain got involved in the process. In fact, the very word "expect" implies that your mind has made an evaluation based on some kind of "evidence" and created an anticipation in response.

Another possibility is that old emotional baggage interferes. Usually these patterns are leftovers from our family. Here is a simplified example: Throughout childhood Sensitive Person "Jane" would reach out to play with her older siblings, only to be bullied and belittled by them. She responded over the years by becoming quieter and by doing their household chores to try to get her siblings to "like" her. All this, only to be rebuffed by them again and again.

Now as an adult, Jane doesn't realize how much she is unconsciously repeating this pattern in her relationships at work. There is a manager who belittles her work, and it sends Jane into a knee-jerk response of withdrawing and taking on extra assignments in attempt to prove her worthiness.

Here is where the pattern gets in the way of intuition. Most people in Jane's department know that the manager is unreasonable and never satisfied, so they do their best to limit contact with her. Jane, on the other hand, keeps approaching her with the expectation that she will now "like" her because of her extra work for the department. All this, only to be rebuffed again and again.

In this example, it's easy to see Jane's pattern and question, "Why would she keep doing that when it doesn't work?" Jane, however, has a different perspective. (It's usually quite a challenge to clearly see one's own dysfunctional patterns.) From Jane's point of view, she says, "I guess I have bad instincts about people. I've run into this over and over. When I interview for a job, it goes well. The manager seems nice, and I expect us to be able to work together well, but then they just don't like me."

Jane continues, "I've even had it happen on dates. Like the last guy I dated seemed really nice at first. I liked him a lot and thought we would get along great. But things started to fall apart. I did everything I could to make the relationship work, but he left me for someone else. I guess I just can't read people."

As you can see from our perspective, Jane's relationship patterns have nothing to do with "reading" people. It is not her empathic sense that is wrong. In fact, Jane isn't tuned in to her intuitive senses at all. The old emotional patterns are a huge barrier that will continue to replay until Jane can see them for what they are. Change requires self-awareness.

I felt it important to give this example because I hear workshop attendees and clients say things like this again and again, "I can't tune in to my intuition," "I'm always wrong about people," and "I tried following my instincts, but it didn't work." We are all in the same boat together. We all have intellectual and emotional barriers to overcome. But what I want you to know is that as a sensitive, empathic person, you *do* have a strong intuitive sense that is ready and willing to help you out at any time. It is there. But sometimes we have to do some digging and cleaning house to unbury it.

Empathic Sensitivity #5
Deep awareness of the emotional energy of domestic and/or wild animals

Humans aren't the only ones vibrating with quantum, emotional energy. Our pets and all animals do as well, in their own way. As an aside, most animals, particularly our domesticated pets, are very empathic, sensitive creatures. They constantly pick up on our emotional energy and react to it. It is a two-way street for many sensitive people and their animal companions.

I have definitely had sensitive clients who know they can naturally "tune in" to their horses or other people's pets and know what the animal is feeling or needing. That isn't necessarily Dr. Dolittle magic. It's empathic communication—a pure form of energetic communication that animals do naturally.

It's well established that all living things on this earth share a surprisingly large amount of genetic code. The genetic code of a little mouse is 88 percent similar to a human's [10] (which is why mice can be used in scientific studies related to human diseases). Since we share so much DNA with our fellow animals, it's not really that much of a leap to consider that we are genetically connected at that quantum, empathic level of existence.

Empathic Sensitivity #6
Feeling stuck with old emotions, particularly after an argument or a negative interaction

"Why can't I let it go?" is a common complaint amongst sensitive people. We often avoid arguments or any unpleasantness because we know it cuts in and sticks like a knife in us for a very long time afterward. This is one of those mysterious aspects of sensitivity that no one can explain really well.

Researchers in the physiological aspects of sensitivity may say it has something to do with the way our brains are more active. More hormones and neurochemicals are released during an argument, and thus that creates a more powerful memory. I'm sure that is part of the reason.

But when a phenomena really can't be explained, that means there is a metaphysical, energetic component. We are missing something in the quantum realm. So I place the "can't shake off negative feelings" experience here in the empathic list. My theory is that when a sensitive

---

10. Carl Zimmer, "Genes are Us. And Them," accessed July 10, 2015, http://ngm.nationalgeographic.com/2013/07/125-explore/shared-genes.

person is on the receiving end of hostility, betrayal, or violence of any kind, there is an empathic, soul reaction of shock—empathic shock. That ethereal impact acts like any other kind of post-traumatic stress disorder—memories of the experience repeat in an unpredictable, yet ever-present cycle.

Luckily, it doesn't have to be that way forever. We'll discuss remedies when we get to chapter 5 about flower essence therapy. There are also many other holistic healing modalities that can relieve this type of thing, such as EFT (Emotional Freedom Technique). I don't teach or use EFT in my practice at this time, but you can learn more about it in books such as *Tapping Into Wellness: Using EFT to Clear Emotional & Physical Pain & Illness* by Kathilyn Solomon.

Empathic Sensitivity #7
Feeling others' physical discomfort or symptoms

Have I mentioned yet that body, mind, and energy are all intertwined? Sorry, I couldn't resist. Physical ailments may manifest in the realm of the body, but they cannot be separated from our emotional and mental energy. Here is an example I've heard more than once at my workshops: "My spouse had a stress headache after work, so I was rubbing his shoulders, when all of the sudden I was overcome with an intense headache myself." Other times the symptom may not be so obvious, as it may come out a little differently once it is filtered through your physical body. But as you can see, this experience of mirroring physical symptoms is basically the same as direct transfer of emotional energy. The energy is just bundled as a physiological experience, rather than an emotional feeling.

Empathic Sensitivity #8
A natural ability to know how to make others feel comfortable

This is an empathic skill that comes in handy. It can't be explained as simply having good people skills. Being empathic means that in many situations we can feel what will make others more engaged, more trusting, and more comfortable.

That can be as simple as noticing the subtle signs during an event that you need to change the seating and move certain people away or together. Or it may be that you know just the right thing to say to someone to bring him out of his shell and invite him into a pleasant conversation.

This is about being highly perceptive and noticing people's subtle signals and body communications. But it is also about that intuitive/empathic lightbulb that goes off, giving you information in each moment about how to create a more peaceful, balanced environment for everyone present.

Empathic Sensitivity #9
Others are drawn to you for advice and may "dump" their worries on you or otherwise take advantage of your kindness

This also is a common theme amongst my workshop participants. "Why do people think it's okay to come over and dump their emotional baggage on me? They leave feeling better, and I'm stuck feeling exhausted." Although we sensitive people often feel like a mess on the inside, we often give others the impression that we are calm, collected, and can deal with anything.

"What? Can't they see that I am stressed, too?" Well, if your friends in question happen to be on the average to less-sensitive end of the scale, then they simply don't notice your subtle signs. Unless you come right out and "dump" as they do, then they think you're doing great.

Let's also consider how empathic energy is a two-way street. Remember we are all quantum and vibrating. We are all sending and receiving emotional energy at all times. You may feel as a sensitive person that you are only on the receiving end, but you broadcast out as well. Your friends will have no idea why, they will simply be drawn to you to help them, and then notice that you somehow always know the right thing to say to make them feel better (see #8).

Another reason that people may take up your time and dump their stuff on you has to do with your own self-concept. Sensitive people have many challenges to their identity and sense of personal value. Depending upon the family you grew up in and other events that shaped you throughout your life, you may feel your only skill is helping other people, or you may feel guilty if you turn someone away who needs help. You might chronically put other's needs before your own. Hence, that is what your friends come to expect of you.

The issue of not being able to say "no" and stand up for the value of one's own space and time is probably the most pervasive theme I see with my sensitive clients. And, unfortunately, I cannot say that it is an easy fix. It comes down to a couple things—learning about your own empathic nature and how it relates to your level of self-respect.

When you are on an airplane, the flight attendant's safety demo always includes, "*Put on your own oxygen mask before assisting others.*" Empathic people are terrible at this. We have a tendency to feel more intensely about other people's suffering than our own. In the context of society as a whole, this is a great quality. We should all step up to help each other. But 99.9 percent of the time is it really that urgent?

In the airplane example, no, it is definitely not more urgent to assist your neighbor first. It is actually far more expedient to take care of your own mask first, then you will have the strength to help both of your neighbors.

But when we are empathic, we sometimes feel the other person's stress, panic, or pain so intensely that it feels like an emergency, even in cases when it really isn't to that person. This happens because empathic sensitivity is pure emotional energy. There is no buffer of intellectual thought or time. There is no explanation of what led up to the person's pain. There is only the emotional energy in its purity in that moment. And that can feel intense, primarily because we were never taught how to be aware of or use our empathic ability. It kind of runs on high all the time until we begin to connect with it more consciously and intentionally.

The other reason empathic people routinely get taken advantage of is an inherent lack of self-importance. Do you really believe that your time is valuable? Do you truly feel that your needs are just as important as everyone else's? Do you ever dare ask your friends or family for assistance, or do you "not want to bother anyone?"

It's a classic catch-22 that plagues empathic people. Deep down inside, whether you are consciously aware or not, you empathically feel a connection to everyone else. That makes empathic people have the reasoning, "I'm not more important than anyone else. We're all in this together." But we often misinterpret that as, "I'm not *as* important as anyone else." "Not *more* important" doesn't have to equal "not *as* important." We can all be equal, and that's where I typically set the bar for empathic people. You are equally as important as every other soul on this earth.

Your brain won't want to believe that. "I'm as important as the president? I don't think so." But that is why your intellect misinterpreted the feeling of that empathic connection in the first place. The intellect only knows the outward roles that define people and their worth. Your empathic sense knows the inherent worth of each person's energy in the collective, and your energy is a vital, important part of that.

If contemplating that doesn't make your friends stop dumping on you so much, try reminding them that you are human too with your own challenges.

Empathic Sensitivity #10
Thinking or problem solving in a creative, outside the box, intuitive way

We've established that sensitive people notice energies and subtle information that others miss. Add into that equation a strong intuition and empathic nature, and you have the ingredients for someone who cannot be content following the status quo. The limitations of the typical state of affairs are way too frustrating for a sensitive person who can easily see options others cannot, and who would prefer to limit unnecessary drama. If you haven't found an environment in which you can be free to express your creative, intuitive ideas, I hope you will very soon. Sensitive people all need that outlet in some way in our lives.

Empathic Sensitivity #11
Deep connection with the meaning of art
and a desire to use it for your own emotional
expression. This also applies to the beauty of nature.

This is one of the great things about being a sensitive person. Where a less-sensitive person may look at a painting and feel nothing, we empathic souls cannot only be inspired with a whole world of messages and meaning from it, we can be overcome physiologically with the joy and beauty of art and nature. It's a meaningful, dynamic way to live.

Many empathic people feel a strong pull to create art in one way or another, such as painting, poetry, crafts, or dance. It's important because creative activity is part of how we encourage our empathic energy to flow and not get so "stuck" within us. So don't think your artistic endeavors are not worthwhile or not "good enough." The same rule applies here as in #9. Your creative expression is equally as important as anyone else's, and it's a healthy, useful mode of empathic communication.

Empathic Sensitivity #12
Inexplicable depression or anxiety
that is unrelated to your life circumstances

We've come full circle, as #12 links in with #1. An empathic person often feels a personal, direct emotional impact from empathically sensing others' "stuff." In this way, empathic feeling can often lead to uncomfortable psychological symptoms such as depression or anxiety, especially when it's not really understood. In other words, when you don't even know empathic ability exists.

Just as the woman who was massaging her husband's shoulders ended up taking on his headache, we sometimes do the same with emotions. Or sometimes we become depressed or anxious from the build-up over time of empathic experiences that we don't understand.

Don't worry. There are ways to modulate all of these experiences. Knowledge is the first key. Now you know that empathic ability exists, and that as a sensitive person you are indeed empathic. This knowledge and awareness changes the game instantly.

Since this acknowledgment of empathic sensitivity is very new to most people, I usually receive this question, "Do empathic people tend to focus on the negative?"

I know it sometimes seems that way when we feel overwhelmed with painful emotions or uncomfortable physical reactions. But the answer is no, it's not that we are focusing on the negative. In regard to our empathic ability, I know that it sometimes seems like we only notice the negative, painful emotions emanating from others. So people sometimes ask me, "Why don't we feel the positive emotions too?" The answer is twofold.

First of all, of course we do also sense people's positive emotions, but sadly, in most situations there simply are more negative emotions present. People at work, school, shopping, or driving are stressed, worried, and preoccupied with their own problems. There just is a lot of unhappiness out there, and that is no reflection upon us as sensitive, empathic people that we seem to feel that more often.

But the other part of the answer has to do with what I call empathic distortion. We grew up in a world that never told us anything about the existence of empathic ability. We had no way to know about it, much less know how to listen to it or use it. The complete neglect of that metaphysical, quantum aspect of who we are leads to distortion. Just think if you were given a saxophone with no lessons and no permission to even read about how the parts of the instrument worked. Your recital would sound pretty distorted as you tried your best to make it work.

Our empathic instrument gets distorted from lack of information and overuse, in a sense. It just keeps on working and becomes louder and louder until we finally pay attention to it. Think about what you hear from speakers when the volume is turned up way too loud. All you hear are distorted tones. The pleasantries of the music are lost. And so it can happen with an empathic sense that is trying to be heard. The empathic distortion smooths out with use of flower essences, which we'll discuss in part 2, and with acknowledgment that we will listen to what our empathic sensitivity is trying to tell us.

So let's do our first guided meditation to acknowledge our empathic sensitivity and let it know that we are open to learning more about it.

Every meditation transcribed in this book is also available in audio file format at www.drkyra.com. I'm providing these written meditation scripts so you can memorize them, record them yourself, or read them aloud to someone else.

. . . .

Empathic Solar Plexus Meditation

In the following meditation, you'll learn to turn your attention away from that place up in your head where you think all day long and focus down into your body where it is much easier to connect with your empathic sense.

Sit comfortably with your back straight and your feet flat on the floor. Begin by taking a slow, deep breath in and out ... Letting go and turning inward. Your breathing becomes a little slower and more relaxed with each breath in and out. Now turn your attention to the top of your head and let all of the muscles in your face and head relax. Let the muscles around your eyes soften ... Your cheeks relax ... Your lips part slightly so that your jaw relaxes.

That relaxation flows down your neck, past your shoulders and all the way down your arms to your hands ... so that your arms feel very heavy, gently relaxing and pulling down your shoulders. The relaxation flows down your back and torso, so that you feel your chest and abdomen expand so easily, effortlessly as you breathe. The heavy relaxation flows down your legs, knees, and all the way down to your feet. You are calm, completely present in this moment right now, peaceful and ready to turn your attention inward.

Now turn your attention to the part of your body that is just below your chest but above your abdomen. This area is called the solar plexus. Below your chest, above your belly, just inside your body there, the solar plexus is an intricate network of nerves that radiates out and connects to every internal organ in your body.

Imagine that for a moment ... a complex network of ganglia and nerves starts there and radiates out to all your important organs.

Now let that image morph. The radiating nerves turn into the rays of a sun. See a bright, glowing sun right there in your solar plexus. Feel the warmth of your sun and its movement as it glows. Notice the colors of your sun, which may be golden or orange but any color that occurs to you is just right. As you tune in to your sun, you may even hear sounds or feel sensations. Everything you notice about your solar plexus sun is right for you.

This sun represents your empathic ability. This is a location in your body where you can connect with your empathic sense. Notice again the warmth, the heat, and the bright power of your sun. Feel fully connected to your internal sun. Connect with your sun. Connect within and know that this is the place where you can communicate with your empathic sense. Again, seeing the bright light, feeling the heat, and sensing the movement as your sun glows.

Fully anchored to this sun, ask it, What do I need to know about my empathic ability? *Anything that occurs to you is just right. You may see a response, hear a reply, or just feel a slight change. Anything you sense is perfect.* What do I need to know about my empathic sense? *Just notice ...*

And now begin turning your attention back to your body. You can leave the glowing sun in place right where it is if you want. Turn your attention back to the chair you are sitting in, and to the sounds in the room around you. Take in a deep, energizing breath. Stretch and move your body a bit, and if you haven't already, open your eyes.

Each person has a unique experience with this meditation. There is nothing in particular that is "supposed" to happen, so don't feel like you did it wrong if you didn't sense a clear, obvious response from your sun. Everyone is different. Some people see a change in their sun when they ask a question, others may hear a reply, and some people simply get a feeling of warmth that seems to grow. Everyone gets clearer feelings with practice. The more you do this meditation, the stronger you will feel a connection to your sun and your empathic sense.

• •

In the next chapter, we'll discuss direct empathic experiences in much more depth, eventually getting to how to transcend and heal the frustrations and discomforts of being empathic in an intellectual world in parts 2 and 3.

CHAPTER 3

More about Empathic Ability

In the previous chapter, we reviewed twelve common ways that empathic sensitivity is expressed. Number 1 was the direct transfer of emotional energy. It's the most mysterious and misunderstood experience empathic people wonder about.

The direct empathic transfer of emotional energy can be the most profound and often the most troublesome type of empathic experience. My story in the introduction is a clear-cut example of this type of empathic experience. My client felt a particular emotional frequency, and I felt the same thing at the same time.

It's not that empathic ability itself is troublesome. Even the direct transfer of emotional energy is really just a neutral form of communication. It's usually useful information to know about someone. Nonetheless, our empathic sensitivity has often led to very uncomfortable symptoms. Why? It's simply because we live in a world that completely denies it could even exist.

Empathic ability is of the spirit/quantum part of our body, mind, and spirit. Yet we live in a world that only acknowledges "body" and just a bit of "mind." What happens then is that people give us "body" and "mind" explanations for what is a "spirit/quantum" phenomenon. That doesn't work.

If you're using the wrong key, it's not going to open the door, no matter how long you stand there fiddling with it. The only "key" that will open the door to understanding and healing of our sensitive, empathic emotional nature is the spirit/energetic key. The other keys don't fit.

This is why so many empathic, sensitive clients have said things to me such as "I feel like I am an emotional sponge. I can't handle being around certain people. Sometimes I am overwhelmed with emotions, and I have no idea how to stop them or even where they are coming from. Yet even when I avoid people, I still feel depressed and overly emotional."

So the key to being more comfortable with your empathic sensitivity isn't about avoiding people and situations (body) and it isn't that anything is irreparably wrong with your emotional psyche (mind)— empathic sensitivity is about embracing our energetic, quantum awareness. Remember in chapter 1 how I said that sensitive people are very perceptive? You might have only been thinking in regard to physical things. That is, that sensitive people are aware of minute details of their environments. But I really meant much more than that. Sensitive people are very perceptive in every realm including the energetic, metaphysical realm of which our empathic sensitivity is always aware.

When this concept is broached in my workshops, it makes my sensitive participants ask these two questions: "Yikes! If I am empathic, how would I know whether a feeling is mine or someone else's?" and "Are you saying you're psychic, and I'm psychic? We're empathically psychic?!?"

To answer the first question about how to discern whether a feeling you're experiencing is yours or empathic, we can look at three tip-offs:

1. The feeling may come on suddenly or out of the blue.
2. The feeling has absolutely nothing to do with the goings-on of your life at that moment.

3. There is a quality to the feeling or the symptom that feels a bit odd or unfamiliar to you.

Now that last one may be subtle, but it is the most important one to eventually learn. It is an acquired skill you'll become more comfortable with as you tune in to your empathic sense. Once we stop blaming ourselves for our emotions and pause the frantic search to figure out "What's wrong with me?," it becomes easier to listen to what our empathic ability is saying, such as with the meditation at the end of the previous chapter.

Now, on to the second question, "We're psychic?" You may notice I have not used the term "psychic" until this point. I've used the words *energetic*, *quantum*, and even *metaphysical*, but for various reasons, "psychic" is a more loaded word. This is partially because the word makes the less-sensitive crowd very uncomfortable. Doctrines of all types have taught people to fear the unknown and have specifically targeted psychic phenomena.

Yet, when we look at the dictionary definition of the word *psychic*, it is neutral. The dictionary definition is: "Lying outside the sphere of physical science or knowledge. Sensitive to nonphysical forces and influences: marked by extraordinary sensitivity, perception, or understanding."[11]

It really isn't that scary of a word, is it? There is much that lies outside the "sphere of physical science or knowledge." Who honestly believes that we humans, in our current state of evolution, know absolutely everything there is to know about ourselves and the world at large? Yes, I know, those people do exist. I'm sure you know at least a couple, and so do I. But even the best scientists out there admit that what we know about ourselves and our world with the tools of physical science is a pittance in contrast to what we don't know.

My point here is that "psychic" simply refers to that which is outside the sphere of physical science. I will admit that the concept stretches

---

11. Merriam-Webster, "Psychic," accessed July 3, 2015, http://www.merriam-webster .com/dictionary/psychic.

most people's comfort zone, as it relates to a person's ability to perceive nonphysical forces and influences.

So, are you psychic? The answer is yes.

If you are sensitive, then yes, you are empathic, which also means you are psychic. If in doubt, check Webster's definition again: "Sensitive to nonphysical forces and influences: marked by extraordinary sensitivity, perception, or understanding."

You may not think of yourself as "extraordinary," but I would disagree. Your sensitivity and ability to perceive and be aware is beyond the limitations of the average level of sensitive perception. It will be easier for you to accept your sensitive strengths when you are no longer embarrassed by your sensitivity or in a panic about the emotional flux of empathic awareness.

A synonym for empathic ability is the term "psychic feeling." You can find a very useful, in-depth discussion of psychic feeling in the book *You Are Psychic!* by Pete A. Sanders. That is yet another book I recommend because it is written by someone who was a trained scientist. Mr. Sanders presents what may seem like "woo-woo" information in a grounded, practical manner, with clear guidance for how to understand and develop one's own psychic sensitivities.

So I am going to say it again: *All sensitive people are empathic and have some level of capacity for psychic feeling.*

Others will disagree with me on this point. I have read many blogs and writings from people with various backgrounds, all with good intentions, I'm sure, on the subject of sensitivity and empathic ability. Some of those blogs have directly stated that empathic people are a subset of the sensitive population, but not all sensitive people are empathic. I disagree 100 percent with that point of view. I base my standing on the observation of thousands of sensitive people who have come to my workshops, have participated in case study research, have written to me, and have been clients.

Let's invoke our mantra again! We are sensitive to *all* vibratory stimuli—body, mind, and spirit—physiological, emotional, and quantum (that which cannot be so easily glossed over with a superficial explanation). Though we humans do try mightily to pull those three components far apart, it cannot be done. Body, mind, and spirit are intertwined. Therefore, I stand by my statement that *all* sensitive people are empathic. We are all impacted by emotional energy. It is part of "spirit" of the body-mind-spirit triad.

Obviously, as with all other aspects of sensitivity, there will be individual differences. We each manifest our sensitivity uniquely. Some of us will naturally be more empathic than others.

Identifying Empathic Feelings

Most sensitive people would not identify themselves as empathic because they simply don't know what it is or how to recognize it. There are a couple reasons that we may not be able to identify our own empathic awareness. One is that we simply aren't looking for it. If you don't even know something exists, that makes it incredibly difficult to notice it. We're taught from an extremely early age that if we feel something, be it physical or a thought or an emotion, then it is obviously our own thing. We own the sensation. Not only are we given no other explanation for it, we are taught that is the *only* explanation for it. If we feel it, we somehow created it.

That's an embedded belief in our individualistic society that is very tough to overcome. It makes sense to our brains. The mind thinks, "I'm sensitive. I feel a ton of stuff all the time, so I guess I'm just overly emotional, too." And we don't have any reason to look into it any further.

Another reason direct empathic transfer can be difficult to identify is that we often don't have the evidence to verify it. In my example of the intense empathic feelings I experienced with a client, I was incredibly fortunate to have been in that role as a psychotherapist. In what other interpersonal situation would I sit with a person for an hour and hear an in-depth description of his feelings? That is exactly how I was able to verify without a doubt that I was empathically feeling his emotions. There was way too much in common for it to be a coincidence.

Usually, though, we don't have the clarification I did in this instance. How would you ever know that you are picking up empathic feelings at your bank job, fast-paced medical office, or with your family that tends to hide emotions? We usually don't know exactly what inner turmoil or even physical discomfort others are experiencing. That makes empathic identification very challenging, especially when our knee-jerk reaction is always to default to, "Whoa, why am I feeling this way? What is wrong with me?" We don't look for empathic clues because no one ever taught us how to do that.

Here's an example of this very thing. In my earlier work on empathy I was more focused on the concept that empathic ability may often be related to sensitive people's tendency toward symptoms such as chronic depression. I myself was a chronically depressed sort of sensitive little kid. There was no good explanation for the type of depression I suffered from. It seemed like it had always been a part of me, a dark, painful force I couldn't control.

I can recall being depressed even as a very young child. Picture a cute little waif of an eight-year-old girl dutifully brushing her teeth before bedtime. She crawls into her bed with her stuffed toys and receives a kiss goodnight from her mother who turns out the lights. The little girl lies awake in bed, staring at the ceiling, and prays, "Please don't let me wake up in the morning." Why would a child have such dark thoughts? Night after night I did. And every morning I was bummed to wake up and find out I was still alive, and to add insult to injury, I had to go to school.

Early in my understanding of empathic ability, I conceptualized it this way: Because I was a sensitive, empathic kid, I was picking up on all sorts of emotions from all sorts of people and places. They were getting all jumbled up within my psyche, causing a confusing emotional landscape, which led to chronic depression. But as it often goes with our theories of the mind, I made it more complicated than I needed to. There was more to the story.

After my previous book was published, my mother read it. She responded to that little story with, "Oh yeah, for a while when you were young, I was so frustrated with my life that I used to cry myself to sleep every night."

I was floored to learn that it was a direct empathic transfer experience after all. I just had no way to know that. I never saw my mother cry, much less had any idea she was crying herself to sleep in the room next to me. I never would have known this if she hadn't told me. Sure, looking back I knew she was unhappy and frustrated, but she was the type of sensitive person who worked hard to appear impervious, and she did a masterful job at it. Thus, she never talked about her own feelings and never showed any emotions where others might see.

I'm sharing this personal story not to say that every emotional experience you have as a sensitive person is empathic. Of course not. We have our own inner emotional river of our personal reactions flowing constantly. Most of our emotions are based solely on the mixture of our own life circumstances, our personality, and our history. On the other hand, not every single emotion we experience is our own stuff.

Nor am I implying that *all* depression has empathic roots. We each have our own history, stressors, and physiology that can lead us to feel depressed for any number of reasons. Rather, all I want you to consider is that empathic sensitivity does exist. It does play a role in who we are as sensitive people, and it does make our emotional landscape more complex than that of someone who is less sensitive.

Thus far, we've been discussing empathic sensitivity from a linear point of view. That's okay because we have to start with the basics. But in order to evolve your empathic ability, it is important to move beyond the "me vs. them" perspective. That is, I have my emotions and you have your emotions and I don't like it when yours leak into mine.

In our culture, we tend to have thoughts that are divisive in two different ways. The first is that we think of ourselves as a separate entity, separate from nature, animals, and every other person on the planet. This is an intellectual construct based on seeing only the purely physical aspects of everything.

The second divisive way of thinking is a habit we all have, and that is judgment. We are quick to categorize every experience as good vs. bad, healthy vs. unhealthy, etc. Even my own use of the terms sensitive vs. less sensitive throughout this book may seem divisionary, even though I don't really mean it that way. Our language is limited, and there is sometimes no other way to succinctly communicate a concept. That said, we still need to be aware of when we are unnecessarily separating and categorizing. Oftentimes, empathic people start out by thinking *It's good for me to feel my own emotions and only my energy. It's bad or unhealthy for me to feel other people's emotional energy.* Truth is, there is no need to label either experience.

Being empathic is actually an opportunity to learn more about yourself as a human being. Empathic feelings are neither good nor bad; they are part of our shared journey. From a quantum perspective, emotional energy is constantly on the move, intermingling amongst all of us.

Emotional Resonance Writing Exercise

The point of this exercise is to demonstrate how we're all in this emotional energy together. This writing exercise will take you several minutes to do thoughtfully, so make sure you have set aside a little bit of time for it. For this activity, please have one or two sheets of paper in front of you. Since this exercise has four steps, I will lead you through an example.

Step 1: At the top of the first page, write an emotional situation that is particularly causing you concern. It should be something that is bothering you quite a bit right now, so that you would really like to figure out a solution for it.

Our example is a fictional woman named Amy who is sad that she isn't spending as much time with her fiancé as she used to. Work and other responsibilities have taken priority, and she is feeling disconnected from her partner. She has begun to lose hope that they are as compatible as she once felt. On the first page she writes: "feeling sad and discouraged about my current relationship."

Step 2: Next, write a list of names of every single person you know of who is also experiencing something similar or that resonates. Your name goes at the end of the list. Some of the names will be people you know well enough that you will feel sure of what they are experiencing. Others on the list may be people that you don't know as well, but you can surmise from things they have said in passing or from other things you have noticed, that they must also be going through a similar emotional situation. If you have difficulty coming up with a list, try getting out of your head. Don't overthink it. Remember to connect with your solar plexus as demonstrated in the meditation at the end of the previous chapter. Write down all of the names that occur to you, even if you aren't sure. This exercise is only for you, and there are no "wrong" answers.

Example: Amy thinks about who else is sad about their relationships. She immediately writes down the name of her friend Lisa who is struggling with ending a relationship with someone who is an alcoholic and doesn't treat her with much respect. Next Amy writes down the name of a coworker, Mike, who is recently divorced and seems lonely.

Amy pauses for a bit and doesn't think she will be able to come up with anyone else for her list, but then her neighbors occur to her. Amy doesn't know her neighbors' names, but she has heard them arguing quite a bit lately. Amy could hear some of what they were saying, and it was obvious that they have strife in their relationship, so Amy wrote "neighbors" third on her list.

Once again Amy thinks she is done, but then remembers her mother talking about Aunt Mary. The family gossip was that Aunt Mary was leaving her husband of thirty-five years to move to Hawaii like she had always wanted to do. Amy wasn't close to Aunt Mary, but could remember seeing her at a family gathering years ago being obviously upset because her husband wouldn't move to a warmer climate. Finally Amy writes herself as the last name on her list.

So Amy's list consists of:

1. Lisa
2. Mike
3. Neighbors
4. Aunt Mary
5. Me

Step 3: Next to each person's name, briefly write what you feel would be the best thing they could do for themselves to change their relationship woes.

1. Lisa—Amy has always felt strongly that Lisa could find someone much better and more deserving of her. So at first Amy thinks she should write "find someone better," next to Lisa's name, but she realizes she needs to consider the bigger emotional picture. When Amy thinks from that perspective, she realizes that Lisa doesn't have strong self-confidence. She doesn't think she deserves anyone better. So Amy writes "Increase self-worth" next to Lisa's name.
2. Mike—At first Amy thinks, *I don't know Mike, how would I know what he should do to feel better?* But then she remembers overhearing other coworkers saying that Mike didn't have any hobbies or interests to get him out to meet new people. Amy writes "Expand interests and hobbies" next to Mike's name.
3. Neighbors—Amy mostly wishes that her neighbors would stop arguing so she wouldn't have to hear them. She writes "Seek counseling" next to number three.
4. Aunt Mary—Amy thinks, *Good for Aunt Mary. She is doing what she has always wanted to do even though her husband wouldn't support her.* So she writes "Be confident that it is okay to make big changes to live the life you want."

Step 4: Before you write a response next to your name, look back over what you wrote for each person on your list, and note which responses would also be helpful to you in your situation.

Remember that Amy is sad and discouraged about her relationship because she feels distanced from her fiancé. They aren't spending as much time together as they used to because of work demands.

Amy thinks for a moment about her situation and realizes that a big part of the reason she is feeling sad and discouraged actually has to do with her job, rather than her relationship. There have been corporate changes at her work, and the environment is not as it once was. Amy's schedule is not as flexible as it used to be, and she leaves work each day feeling tired. She was discouraged because she and her fiancé were no longer doing fun activities, but Amy realized that really was due to them both being too tired at the end of the workday.

She looks back at #1. Her feeling about Lisa was that she would benefit from increasing her self-worth. When Amy looks at it again, she realizes that her own self-worth took a big hit at work when the company was reorganized and she did not receive a promotion she expected. Amy then realized she had let that drop in self-esteem affect everything in her life, even how she was relating to her fiancé.

#2. Amy wrote "expand interests and hobbies" for Mike. Amy recognized that this could also apply to her situation. She had been meaning to try new activities, such as yoga, to help her deal with her work stress, but she hadn't done it yet.

#3. "Seek counseling" was what Amy had written in regard to her neighbors' arguments. With this Amy sighed, and she remembered that she had a passing thought recently to make an appointment with her old therapist for career counseling.

#4. And lastly Amy wrote "Be confident that it is okay to make big changes to live the life you want" when thinking about Aunt Mary. Amy admitted to herself that she was putting off doing what she really wanted, which was a career change, and that was the biggest part of the discouragement she was feeling.

So for herself, Amy wrote "Talk with my fiancé about my desire to change my career and how we can change our lifestyles to have the energy and time to have fun again."

Amy wondered a bit if she was empathically sensing any of the frustration or sadness from anyone on her list, but she realized that in this particular instance it really didn't matter. Just by recognizing the emotional energy they all had in common, it helped Amy see her own emotional response from a different, clearer perspective.

When you do this exercise, you may be surprised by how many people you can list who are feeling something similar to you. We are all going through the human experience. Please remember that this activity is solely for you to see the resonance of emotional energy amongst everyone on the list. This exercise allows you to think in a new way about the shared emotional energy of most situations. It is not for you to share with the people on your list, so do not worry about writing anything that may not be perfectly accurate.

• •

Your experience with the activity may be different from Amy's. You may or may not feel as connected to every response you wrote, as Amy did. And you may realize that you are indeed picking up empathically on someone else's feelings, exacerbating your own similar emotions. In either case, this exercise gives you clarity about the emotions you are experiencing, and what you can do to best heal and move forward. When you do that, it is much less likely that you will be overwhelmed empathically by anyone on your list, as you will have changed the resonance of your energy.

That's a very important point: *We will be most affected empathically by emotional energy that has a similar resonance to our own.* This is one key reason why self-development is vital for empathic people. The more we heal and understand ourselves, the less impacted we are by other people's painful emotions. It is no more complicated than a resonance of energy.

So let's take a look again at my story in the introduction. You may ask, "In your example, you described Dan's thoughts as things that were not applicable to your own life, so how is that a resonance of energy?"

True, the specific feelings that Dan had about being a hopeless failure were not thoughts that I was having in any way, and that gave me a tip-off that perhaps the feelings were not mine. But there still was a resonance of energy. Throughout my life, I've had a tendency toward depression, similar to Dan's recurrent melancholy. Although I did pick up on people's anxiety once in a while in the earlier stages of my empathic journey, I was much more likely to be impacted by other people's depression.

I've also made the statement that every empathic emotion we experience is an opportunity to learn something about ourselves. Our empathic experiences are often communication from our own inner wisdom about what we need to clear or heal for our own healing path or something else we need to know. So what did I learn from Dan? That one was pretty straightforward. I learned from him that I was very empathic, and that was something that I definitely needed to learn about myself.

Now when I realize I am picking up on anyone else's uncomfortable or painful emotions, it is usually a sign to me that I have slipped a bit and have allowed myself to fall back into unhelpful patterns. There is always a resonance to the empathic emotions that helps me clearly see how what I'm feeling is detrimental to my own energy. Once I realize that and shift as needed, the empathic connection dissipates.

This is why I created the Emotional Resonance Writing Exercise (see page 54) to help you identify that resonance of energy and figure out how you can move beyond it. I call this process "raising our vibration."

Empathic Protection vs. Raising Our Vibration

Another concept that seems appropriate but can actually be more limiting than helpful is the idea of psychic protection. Think of the word "protection" and what occurs to you? A wall? A fortress? A shield in battle? "Protection" has a tone to it that implies that something harmful needs to be kept out. Otherwise why would you need protection? It also implies a certain weakness. That is, the other energy is stronger, so I need reinforcements.

Now I am not saying at all that anyone has ever done anything wrong by using the word *protection* or by writing a book about psychic protection. As I said earlier, our language is limited, and sometimes certain words have to be used to get a point across. But, please consider with me that we humans are evolving. We need to continue moving away from us vs. them and toward collective compassion and cooperation. This is most true in the energetic realm of empathic development.

Think instead about raising your vibration. Your energy becomes healthier, happier, and lighter and that makes you naturally less impacted by the darker, heavier energies. Remember resonance. As you raise your vibration, you more easily move away from the heavier, painful energies. There is no attraction. And, instead, your balanced energy will find resonance with fellow positive, healthy people.

For most of us, this is a never-ending healing self-journey kind of process that has its ups and downs, but it is definitely worth the effort. I've been consciously working on it for going on twenty years and expect the healing journey to continue to my last breath in this life. And the more I continue this lifestyle, the less it becomes work and the more it simply becomes an interesting, rewarding way to live. I want you to know that this is how your empathic sensitivity can evolve— from something confusing and uncomfortable to a connection with your own inner wisdom.

I know all too well, though, that empathic sensitivity can be troublesome in the beginning stages of our awareness of it. It takes a while to learn what it is trying to teach us about ourselves.

If you are currently feeling overwhelmed and confused by your empathic ability, it can be a very distressing and isolating experience. Therefore, I want to give you as many resources as I can to help you in this book. Another perspective is always helpful. I felt it important to give you an example of someone else who has also learned to be comfortable with her empathic ability in a very positive way over the course of her life. When considering who I knew that fit that description, I knew I should ask Molly Sheehan from Green Hope Farm, a flower essence manufacturer. Molly describes her life as an empath in a very down-to-earth, honest way. She has contributed a summary in Appendix A: Another Perspective on Being Empathic.

Let's move on to part 2 of this book where you'll learn that no matter how uncomfortable or confusing your sensitivities may be right now, they are fluid and changeable. You can evolve how you experience your sensitivity. I know this because I've come a very, very long way since the days of my empathic overwhelm as a young psychotherapist. The key steps have been: trusting my own instincts about my experiences; looking beyond conventional, mainstream approaches to sensitivity; and a willingness to continually walk the path of self-compassion, clearing, and healing. You too, can learn to live primarily from the positive strengths of your sensitivity. Creativity, intuition, and empathic ability can provide you with meaning and insight on a daily basis.

With new information and tools, you can begin this process by recalibrating your sensitivity to a much more comfortable setting. Let's talk first about how sensitivity is changeable.

Part II

Sensitive Recalibration

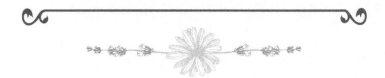

CHAPTER 4

Sensitivity Is Changeable

Yes, I said it, folks. Your sensitivity and the way it manifests for you physically, emotionally, and energetically is changeable. Say what? "I've been sensitive my entire life. Won't I always be that way?"

Well, sure, you'll always be a sensitive person. But the discomforts associated with being sensitive don't have to stay exactly the same. Remember that the definition of sensitive is not "an uncomfortable person." It is an "aware and perceptive person." Discomforts emerge because of societal things such as disbelief of empathic ability, a lot of drama and negativity in our environment, and our willingness to believe that something is wrong with us.

So, to be clear, this chapter is not about changing the core nature of who you are as a sensitive person. Believe me, a thousand times I've heard, "So I'm empathic? Great! Tell me how to turn it off!" Sorry, there is no off switch for who you are, but we can dial it down a bit by redefining ourselves in more positive ways; learning more about all the different ways we are sensitive in body, mind, and energy; accepting our own self-worth; and using self-development to clear out unhealthy patterns and limiting beliefs.

You can eventually be both sensitive and pretty comfortable. You are not doomed to always be overwhelmed by the world.

These days there are a lot of people writing about sensitivity, and that is fantastic! Sensitivity is finally being recognized as okay. Attempts are being made to understand sensitivity from a scientific perspective. But, at this time, most of the writings I have seen continue to imply that we are hardwired for whatever level of sensitivity we currently experience, and all we can expect is to continue that through our lives. Many authors suggest maintenance for how to take care of ourselves so that we don't make our discomfort any worse than it already is.

I personally believe that is an unfortunate and unnecessary way to view our sensitive tendencies. I give other researchers and authors their due respect, though. When conceptualizing sensitivity from a purely physiological or conventional viewpoint, it does seem permanent in nature. We just are what we are—easily overwhelmed and depleted by life.

But add in energy, empathic awareness, and quantum ways of thinking, and we become much more than just physically and emotionally sensitive. The definition of who we are shifts. A sensitive person is someone who can enjoy the nuances of everything life has to offer—physical, emotional, and energetic. If you would allow me to go poetic for a few paragraphs, I will elaborate on this statement.

We exist full-bore in all the sensations, feelings, and energy that we sense and that we create in turn. We perceive it all. We don't miss a thing, and why would we want to? Like a young child enamored with the astoundingness of all there is to see and do in the big, wide world, we can encounter something new and interesting every day. Why? Because we *notice*.

The details don't escape us, and that is where treasures are found. The subtlest energies provide impetus for an intuitive thought and a kind gesture that someone needs just at that very moment. We make the world a better place, a warmer place.

Our awareness goes beyond the boundaries most people impose on the world. In fact, we are examples in action that there is no such thing as a hard boundary anywhere. Not between people, not between the environment and our own bodies, not even between our inner feelings and the outer world. So we must stop listening to people who tell us we need to build walls and reinforce our boundaries. Doing so only hurts us because it tries to take away our primary gift: *feeling the truth*. One of the worst things I witness sensitive, empathic people do is try to put themselves into a fortress. I understand the desire. I did the same thing for much of my life. But, all things in moderation. Yes, basic boundaries are healthy in order to define our identity vs. someone else. I'm not saying you should remove all boundaries and become enmeshed with everyone else. This is instead about *flow*. Trying to create impenetrable boundaries in the physical and emotional planes basically just doesn't work. The main thing it accomplishes is to make your world smaller.

We've established that even if you try to maintain distance, withdraw from situations, and create boundaries, you've done nothing to change the fact that you are empathic, which defies time, space, or any other seeming barrier. But you can change the way your sensitivity flows, the way you interpret it, and your irritation with it by having more compassion for yourself.

Here's another way to conceptualize flow rather than boundaries. I think of dolphins as kind of like sensitive people. We both live in two very different worlds. Dolphins live primarily in the sea, but they have to come up frequently with their heads out of the water, dependent on breathing air to survive.

Sensitive people exist primarily in a world we'll call "the sea," in which we perceive the nuances all around us, in which we are energetically connected to everything, and which is balanced in the way we like (without excessive stimuli of noise, smells, anger, etc.). But we frequently have to stick our heads into the "air," which is the less-sensitive day-to-day world where we have to work, shop, and generally interface with society.

The dolphin doesn't even think of creating boundaries between its home in the sea and the surface world above. It would suffocate if it did. The dolphin has to be able to flow seamlessly between its two worlds. And so do we.

We may be more comfortable in the sea of sensitive familiarity, but in order to survive (i.e., earn money, buy food, have at least a few friends and associates) we have to spend a lot of time in the air. So how do we become comfortable flowing between the sea and the air?

The first, most important step is to reframe everything you've ever been told about who you are as a sensitive person. If you are to become more comfortable physically, you must also become more comfortable in your mind and in your heart about who you are. Doesn't it make sense that if you are to change how your body reacts, you must also change how you feel about yourself?

I am not saying you've ever done anything wrong to feel animosity toward your sensitive nature. And I am most certainly not saying that you have done anything to cause your physical sensitivities. All I am saying is that we sensitive people exist in all realms quite equally. Let's add a fourth realm for this discussion to be more accurate. We exist very fully in all these realms of being: the physical, the mental, the emotional, and the etheric. If we've been beaten down through life experiences in one realm, then we'll feel the effects in all the realms. If we begin to consciously uplift ourselves in one or more realms, then we also will feel the uplifting, healing effects in all the realms.

This falls under the "raising our vibration" process described in the previous chapter. It's easiest for us to start on the mental plane where we can start noticing what thoughts we allow ourselves to have. Notice if you are thinking any of these types of thoughts, and if so, how often:

- I'm too sensitive.
- No one else is like me.
- I'll never be strong like other people.
- I'm mad at my body (or emotions) for being so sensitive.
- I have to hide my sensitivity because others will think I'm weak.
- I'd rather put my own needs aside than get into an argument.
- I can't enjoy life because of my sensitivity.

You get the picture here. I would imagine that just by reading these statements, you felt a dark, depressing sort of energy. I know I do. So what happens when you think these things to yourself over and over throughout the day? It traps you in a vicious cycle of contempt for your sensitive nature.

. . . .

Changing Self-Defeating Thoughts Writing Exercise

For this exercise, keep a small pad of paper with you all day, or if you know how to keep notes on your phone, that is fine too. Every single time that you think a self-defeating or limiting thought, especially about your sensitivity, write it down. If you have trouble maintaining that level of self-observation or just forget to write some down, do it again the next day.

At the end of the day, review your list and write down more helpful, positive alternatives. For example, if you thought, "I'm too trusting. I always get taken advantage of," write an alternative such as, "I have strong, accurate instincts about people" or "People treat me with respect."

Then for the rest of the week keep your new list with you and try to replace your previous limiting thoughts with the new alternatives. The old, self-defeating thoughts are a habit. It takes practice to consistently interrupt the old thoughts and replace them with the new affirmations. But if you stick with it, eventually the old, habitual thoughts will start to fade. When you are aware, then you can stop what for many sensitive people is a never-ending cycle of self-defeating thoughts. Thus you begin to have more compassion and kindness toward yourself.

. . . .

So what else do I mean when I say that sensitivity is changeable? What I mean is that it is fluid. Think about how different we are at different times. How differently do you feel when you are coming down with a cold vs. the relief when you have finally successfully completed a big project at work? Think about how you feel when you are aggravated with one of your kids vs. the peacefulness that can encompass you when you go to your favorite beach or lake, for example.

Now think about how different your sensitivities are in all these various situations. All your sensitivities will be ramped up and agitated when you are ill or stressed. At those times you may suddenly realize that noises are bothering you more. You have to take out the smelly trash right now! Or that joking comment that was fine last week is now bothering you and bringing up painful memories. On the other hand, when you are feeling very healthy and strong, it's likely that your physical sensitivities will be less pervasive, and you'll be able to think clearly about what is best for your own health.

A common thing sensitive people think is something along the lines of, "Ughh, I'm so sensitive! Why does this have to bother me so much?" Think about what you are telling yourself when you are frustrated and say that. You are essentially agreeing that you are "too sensitive" and it is always that way. I'd like you to shift the self-blaming energy of that comment to focus instead on the fluidity of the situation. What can be changed?

There are situations that make us feel frustrated with our sensitivities. Examples include: the smell of someone's deodorant or hair products make you feel ill, someone's remark in a meeting hurts your feelings, or your son's music leaves you feeling very unsettled and irritable. Remember we don't want to beat ourselves up about having the sensitive reaction. Instead of asking "Why do I have to feel this way?" Instead, we ask "Is this something that I have to endure in my environment or can it be changed?"

A bad habit many sensitive people have is defaulting to tolerating the status quo. That is, believing they need to endure all the annoyances in their lives. Other people's perfume at the theater, the neighbor stopping by to chat too frequently, or a lack of raises at work ... these are examples of things that sensitive people often politely endure, but there is no reason to. Yet we often do it to the sacrifice of our own peace of mind and health. So, instead of tolerating something that agitates you, ask "Is this something that I absolutely have to endure?"

If your answer is yes: First stop and reconsider. Is there really absolutely nothing that can change in the situation? Most circumstances are not fixed. They can be changed somehow, even if just a little. It's often our way of looking at the situation that makes it seem un-changeable. For example, maybe the music your son loves is agitating you more and more these days. You want to give him the freedom to listen to music he likes and pursue his interests, but you can hear it, it's grating on your nerves, and you are becoming more irritable. Your reaction has been to tolerate it, thinking, *He only listens to it for a while. I can deal with it for a couple hours.*

But why tolerate something on a regular basis that takes you off-center? A point to remember is that our sensitive nervous systems re-act to stimuli very strongly. After that reaction causes a spike, it often takes our nervous systems a long, long time to recede back to baseline. It's much better to avoid the disturbance in the first place, rather than deal with the recovery period.

So let's reconsider Mom's approach to her son's music. She has felt it important to allow him some freedom and to show respect for his in-terests, and she has decided she needs to tolerate his music. In her ap-proach to this issues, she has not considered the compromises that ex-ist—headphones for her son, playing ambient noise such as nature sounds that might block out her son's music, asking him to turn down the volume while she is home with chances for him to listen at a louder volume when she is out working in the yard or at a yoga class, having her son listen to his music down in the basement where the sound won't travel as much. In other words, there are actually many options that change the particulars of the situation. It is not disrespectful nor inconveniencing her son to ask him to slightly alter his habits for Mom's comfort.

This was a concrete example, but the same rules apply to issues such as asking to be compensated fairly at work or asking someone to stop making joking, but hurtful comments. There generally are more op-tions available to change the situation than we think. Talking to some-one else with a different viewpoint can often help us see the options we aren't seeing.

But if your yes is an absolute, firm yes that nothing at all can be done to change a situation that is aggravating your sensitivities, then here is the next question to ask: "What is your sensitive reaction telling you about yourself?" For example, is there something very unhealthy for you in your environment? Or is something else setting off your sensitivities that is "hidden," like a food intolerance? Or is it time to make a big change to leave the situation you are in?

. . . .

What Can Be Changed?
Brainstorming Exercise

Take out a blank piece of paper and write down a current situation that is exacerbating your sensitivities. This should be something resembling the previous examples that makes you feel frustrated and unsure how to handle the situation.

Now brainstorm and write down every possible way the situation could change so that it is no longer so agitating to your sensitivities. This is brainstorming, so that means you let the ideas flow without judging them. You may write down possibilities that are very unlikely to happen. That's okay. Write down everything that occurs to you. That is how you'll eventually happen upon something you had never considered before. If you get stuck, you may need to take a little break and then come back again later.

Once you have written all of the ideas that occur to you, go back and look over your list and circle the ones that are the most likely options that you will actually do.

. . . .

This discussion has been about reducing our tendency toward self-blame for our sensitive reactions. But, I know, that sometimes you may truly feel like your sensitivities are far more uncomfortable than warranted given the situation. The next chapter discusses a little-known holistic approach that can actually recalibrate your sensitive reactions by working with your etheric energy. The biggest key to change for sensitive people is through the door of the energetic part of who you are. It is the most unfamiliar part of yourself and, ironically, the most expansive. The energetic part of the body-mind-spirit triad is the most dynamic and flexible. This quantum part of ourselves is the fastest to embrace change and in a lot of ways the easiest to communicate with ... as long as you have some help to get started.

That help is exactly what I'll be introducing you to in the next chapter. We'll discuss one type of energetic approach that works perfectly for sensitive people to help us recalibrate ourselves in body, mind, and spirit.

CHAPTER 5

Introduction to Flower Essence Therapy

In this chapter, I'll introduce an unconventional healing therapy called flower essences. Flower essences are extremely useful for helping us recalibrate our sensitivity and raise our vibration.

What Are Flower Essences?

Flower essences are wonderful gifts from nature that deliver the energetic vibration of flowers directly to us to help us heal in a myriad of ways. They are a little-known remedy. Most people have never heard of them. That's because flower essences are vibrational medicine on the quantum level. They are made only from the flowers of various plants and trees. These unique remedies help us transform, recalibrate, and heal, especially in emotional and energetic ways.

Please note that flower essences are *not* the same as essential oils. During my workshops I spend time explaining in-depth exactly what flower essences are and how they are made. Then a participant will ask a question about them and refer to them as "oils," as if I had been talking for the past thirty minutes about essential oils in aromatherapy. I get it, people like aromatherapy. It smells nice. It's understandable. But there is a big difference between the two.

To make an essential oil, a large amount of plant matter is harvested and distilled down into a concentrated liquid form. It's very physical. That makes sense to our brains, and it's easy to envision.

Flower essences, on the other hand, are not a comfortably familiar item at all. Flower essences are water-based remedies that have no smell. They are primarily used by putting their drops in water and drinking the water throughout the day. They heal with energy, not with physical matter. This is a quantum way to think about healing, and so folks have a tough time accepting what they are. You've got to let your mind relax and let go of judgment to ever be able to understand what flower essence are. It's best to just let the information flow in and decide that you'll try to figure it all out later.

So what is the flower of a plant? Let's think about that for a moment. What does the flower represent? How is it different from the rest of the plant? Let's do a quick visualization. Think about your favorite flower. Now see it out in a garden or in a meadow. Notice how beautiful and maybe fragrant the flower is. It's very different from the rest of the plant, and it's only there some of the time.

The flower of a plant is the pinnacle of the core energy of the plant. The flower is the embodiment of beauty and creativity. It also is dynamic, quite unique from every other kind of flower, and it will ultimately lead to how the plant reproduces. The flower is the sensitivity, the expansive power, and the creativity of the plant. In essence, it is the soul of the plant.

The flower has healing qualities, just like the other parts of the plant do. But whereas the roots and leaves tend to offer healing for specific physical ailments, such as wound healing or soothing an upset stomach, the flower essence offers the plant's particular healing qualities in the energetic realm.

How are flower essences made? Here's where it really becomes clear why I recommend flower essences so highly for sensitive people. Flower essences are traditionally made by respectfully harvesting the flowers, placing them in water, and then providing the right time and environment for the healing energy of the flower to be transferred to the water. Then that water is bottled in small dropper bottles, so that we can take the remedy internally or use it topically.

Flower essences cannot be made by just anybody. They can only be made by an intuitive, sensitive person. There is no other way it can be done. Flower essences require an empathic nature lover who can commune with the plant with utmost respect. The flower essence creator must be able to feel the very subtle energies of the flowering plant to know all the details: when is the right time to pick it, what healing qualities it offers (especially if creating a new essence from a never-before-used plant), and tips for how people should use it.

Flower essence manufacturers do what they do because they love nature, and because they feel called to do this healing work. Flower essences must be made with sensitivity and with love. They will not work any other way. I would be severely remiss if I did not include them in this book because they are an optimal healing method for sensitive people. It's the sensitive part of the plant, made by a sensitive person, offering deep emotional and energetic healing that will be most easily felt by sensitive people.

Flower essences are remedies directly from that sensitive, empathic realm. The healing water in those little flower essence bottles reverberates to our depths of sensitivity, encouraging us to shift and change in beneficial ways that we did not know were even possible.

It may help some of you to know that my appreciation for flower essences is due solely to the incredible transformations I have experienced and witnessed. They provide empathic, emotional, and energetic support that sneaks past intellectual barriers, allowing us to clear, heal, and shift in profound ways. Flower essences ease the discomfort of being sensitive. Period.

Their effectiveness is the only reason I am such a fan. I don't own a flower essence company. I don't profit in any way, shape, or form from your purchase of flower essence remedies from any brand. So know that I'm neutral. I share this information with you as a fellow sensitive person because I know what flower essences can do for you.

Why Flower Essences?

Despite my use of the word "healing," I am not saying we sensitive people need to use this remedy called flower essences to fix what is broken about us. Flower essences are an ally in our evolution. They are a friend from Mother Earth, a friend who understands precisely who we are as sensitive people and gifts us with the type of energy that has been lacking in our lives. Just like a good friend who brings over a nice, hot, comforting meal when we are stressed out, flower essences are the friend who brings just exactly the energy we've been looking for when we most need it.

In my workshops, I often receive two questions about flower essences. The first is, "Do we really need to take them?" In short, yes. If you really want to recalibrate your sensitive reactions, transcend persistent emotional discomfort, and evolve along in your personal healing journey, then yes, flower essences will offer a significant piece that I have not found in any other healing modality.

The second is really the same basic question: "Isn't there anything else I can do instead, like visualization?" With this question, I understand that the person is reticent to take a remedy or may be suspect of such a metaphysical creation. I've noticed among workshop participants that there is a strong contingent of people who believe that if they could just find the right visualization—a mirror, a door, a screen—they will have successfully found their internal boundary enhancer, and all would be better from then on.

Meditation and mindfulness are important components of sensitive evolution that we'll be discussing in chapter 7, but one simple visualization is not going to make a difference. That's because there are two flaws to the hope for a boundary-enhancing visualization. The first is buying into the conventional societal belief that we should be able to use the strength of our mind to fix this "problem." We search for an intellectually logical visual, and we assume that should do the trick. If you've read the chapters leading up to this point, you should already be able to answer why this approach misses the mark. We are sensitive because we exist in much more than just the intellectual realm. An approach that comes primarily from the intellectual realm isn't going to harmonize with us in the ways that we truly need.

The second flaw has to do with boundaries. If you read all of the previous chapters then you've gotten enough information about the reframing boundaries concept. Fortifying boundaries is not the most successful approach, nor is it the ultimate answer to evolve your sensitivity. Again, it's an intellectual idea that is only useful or effective up to a point. After that, we have to focus more on flow, evolution, and approaching our sensitivity from the realm that has been most ignored—the energetic realm where the most dramatic change can more easily occur.

Are there other healing approaches that may be useful for you? Of course, there are many to choose from: EFT, Reiki, hypnotherapy, pranic healing, acupuncture, yoga, and on and on. But there is no reason that flower essence therapy shouldn't also be included in the things you choose to support your evolution. If you really do not want to ingest a remedy, please refer to my How to Use section (see page 83) in which I discuss topical and visual uses of flower essences, no ingestion required.

My #1 Flower Essence Recommendation: Yarrow

Now let's move on to discuss the essence that I've seen provide the most profound healing for sensitive people. Yarrow is a common plant that easily grows wild or cultivated in gardens throughout temperate climates. Its Latin name is *Achillea millefolium*, which refers to its very finely dissected, lacy leaves. Yarrow's flower head is also complex. It is made of many tiny flowers all compacted into a larger flower head. Yarrow is a powerful herbal remedy that has been used for centuries as a woundwort, meaning that it heals cuts and wounds.[12]

We've danced around the concept of plants having body, mind, and spirit much the same as we do. Yarrow is the perfect example of a

---

12. Clare Hanrahan, Gale Encyclopedia of Alternative Medicine, "Yarrow," accessed January 2, 2014, http://www.encyclopedia.com/topic/yarrow.aspx.

plant that clearly exhibits that. It has a very strong, clear history as an herbal healing remedy. We'll call that the "body" part of its personality, the way that it heals our bodies. You'll see that there is an obvious parallel between how yarrow is used as an herbal remedy (body) and the energy it has as a flower essence (spirit).

I mentioned above that yarrow has been used for centuries as a woundwort, a plant that was known to heal wounds, particularly deep, bleeding cuts. It was used for such purposes for warriors, who would carry yarrow in a pouch with them into battle. If a soldier received a deep laceration, he would hopefully be lucky enough to be able to move and apply the yarrow leaves to the wound, or someone else would do it for him. The yarrow had three healing actions that would most likely save the warrior's life:

- It staunched the bleeding, so he would not bleed to death.
- It was antimicrobial, so the wound would not become infected.
- And, maybe most amazingly, yarrow promoted the skin to knit back together and heal neatly with reduced scarring.

This information about yarrow isn't just folk tale. Herbalists still frequently use yarrow for its powerful healing properties today. You can learn more in *The Book of Herbal Wisdom: Using Plants as Medicines* by herbalist Matthew Wood.

Most of us who have studied herbalism even a little bit have had our own injuries and chances to test out yarrow to see if it really does heal wounds that well. I can attest from my own fall while holding a glass bottle and subsequent deep cut on my hand, that yarrow does indeed do everything the warriors entrusted it to do.

So that is what the leaves of the yarrow plant do. But what happens when a sensitive, intuitive person uses only the yarrow flower and makes it into a flower essence? Very similar actions, but the healing is expressed in that energetic spirit realm of who we are. So let's review those three actions again, from the flower essence perspective.

Yarrow staunches bleeding. How does the energetic corollary help sensitive people? There's a reason empathic people are called "bleeding hearts." We often give too much of ourselves and deplete our energy. Yarrow flower essence helps us learn how to reel that back in so we don't exhaust our energy stores.

Herbal yarrow inhibits the growth of microorganisms. Flower essence yarrow does the same type of action by increasing the vibration of our energetic body, helping it naturally repel that which is unhealthy and unwanted.

Yarrow promotes wounded skin to knit back together cleanly, with minimal scarring. All of us sensitive people have incurred empathic emotional wounds throughout our lives. Flower essence yarrow heals the lingering effects of those wounds, in essence repairing our etheric body, helping us feel stronger and more energetically intact.

Flower essence yarrow gives sensitive people something we do not find elsewhere in our day-to-day world, and that is radical acceptance of our empathic sensitivity. We are able to perceive and feel energy—from other people, from places, and from electromagnetic sources. Since we were repeatedly taught in our world to dismiss these feelings, we've had no way to understand, much less manage, this energetic sensitivity. Yarrow pushes the reset button, so that we can start fresh again with new knowledge and awareness.

My clients and workshop participants over the years have reported the following types of responses to yarrow flower essence:

• Feeling less overwhelmed in general

• Better sleep

• Less annoyance with things that used to bother them before (e.g., the neighbor using his weed whacker, the sound of utensils hitting the plates at dinner, coworker noises in the next cubicle)

• Improved clarity about empathic emotions; that is, knowing what is their own vs. what is not

The flower essence that I've been describing is from the white yarrow flower. Several US flower essence manufacturers have white yarrow essence: Flower Essence Services (FES), Alaskan Essences, Featherhawk Essences, Freedom Flowers, and Green Hope Farm.

Some manufacturers make yarrow essence from different colored yarrows (pink, golden, red, lavender), and each color has a slightly different focus to its healing energy. The manufacturers all have great websites and books with detailed descriptions. Some of the manufacturers are listed in appendix B of this book, including flower essence companies in other countries.

When you read the yarrow descriptions from different manufacturers, you'll notice that each one is just a little bit different. That's okay. A flower essence is not chemical medicine that has just one definition. Rather, a flower essence remedy is a quantum creation born from the interface between the soul of the flower and the spirit of the person making it. From that perspective, it makes sense that each manufacturer has its own slightly unique take on it.

When you read the descriptions, you'll also notice that some of the manufacturers use the word "protection." If you'll recall from chapter 3, I stated that it is more useful for us to replace the word "protection" with the ideas of recalibration and raising our vibration, thus reducing our resonance with unhealthy or painful energies. But I am not the word police. I'm not going to exclude essences that have beneficial energy just because of one word. Just as we all do, the flower essence manufacturers have to use succinct wording that will communicate a concept to the most people possible. Eventually, more and more people will understand energetic resonance. Until then, just mentally replace "protection" with "recalibration" when you see it.

Learning about Other Flower Essences

Once you start learning a little bit about flower essences, you'll find out that there are thousands of them in addition to yarrow! Each and every flowering plant on the earth has its own healing contribution to lend to us. I love to think about that—each and every flower I see when I am out on a walk or visiting a garden has its very own personality and healing energy that it is just waiting to share with humanity. There are flower essences that help us heal the trauma from abuse, ease differing types of depression and anxiety, soothe heartbreak and grief, get better in tune with our intuition, and on and on and on.

Flower essences work so well for sensitive people because we are naturally receptive to their healing frequencies. There is this huge toolkit from nature in existence to help you along your path no matter what your individual circumstances may be.

How to Use Flower Essences

Flower essences are energetic, vibrational remedies. They work from the realm of quantum energy. This is a new concept for most of us. In our world, we are used to using medications that are forcefully physiological and chemical.

Flower essences are very different. They are subtle and yet can have very profound effects. Why? Because they work *with* our own energy and innate wisdom. Even when we aren't consciously aware of it, there is always a part of ourselves, deep down somewhere, that knows exactly what we need to shift and what we need to heal. Flower essences work in cooperation with that innate wisdom.

Chemical medicines on the other hand, though sometimes helpful and needed, work by forcing a physiological response. It's no wonder, then, that sensitive people often experience side effects and uncommon reactions to chemical medications. Our highly reactive and aware systems don't appreciate a giant shove when a gentle nudge is sufficient. This review is to remind you how different flower essences are from the medicines we are used to taking. Therefore, flower essences can be used in several ways, all quite different from chemical medication.

Internal Usage of Flower Essences

Flower essences are liquid remedies in a dropper bottle. Since the liquid is only a delivery mechanism for the quantum energy, a very small amount is all that is needed per dose.

I prefer that my clients put three to four drops in water and drink that water throughout the day and evening. But most people want to know numbers and times, so the standard dosage for flower essences is four drops, four times per day. The point is that the more often you expose your energy to the healing catalyst of flower essence energy, the quicker and more effectively you can begin to feel its effects.

Some flower essence instructions may say that the drops can be put directly under the tongue. That's okay, but as I stated above, I have found it much better for people to take the remedies in water. It keeps your dropper clean, you can see how many drops you are using, and the water is a carrier that helps the flower essence energy gently meld with your own.

Some brands preserve the flower essence liquid in the traditional way with brandy. Other brands are preserved with other things, such as vinegar, glycerin, or a plant called red shiso. If you don't like the idea of alcohol in the remedy or think you might not react well to it even in minute amounts, then you will want to choose from one of the several flower essence manufacturers that do not use alcohol in their preparations.

The most widely distributed brands that are available through your local co-op or herb shop are Flower Essence Services (FES) and Bach Flower Remedies. Both of these brands use the traditional brandy method. If you want to use those because of the ease of buying them locally or from a familiar retailer, realize that the alcohol content will be extremely diminished when just a few drops are put into a full glass of water. If you want the alcohol to evaporate entirely, add the drops to hot tea or to hot water, which you could then allow to cool for use throughout the day.

External Use of Flower Essences

The essences can also be used topically, rather than internally. Flower essences present us with a resonance of quantum healing energy. So there is no unbreakable rule that they have to be taken internally. It also affects our energy, particularly the most sensitive of us, to apply the drops to our skin or to simply hold the bottle.

You'll notice that some manufacturers offer spray bottles of flower essence mixtures, often combined with aromatherapy. The flower essence drops can be put in baths, foot baths, or mixed in with your daily lotion. Some of my clients like to purchase a tiny bottle necklace (these can be found online by searching for bottle pendant or necklace) and put their flower essence drops in the bottle pendant. Then they have that energy with them all the time they're wearing it. That's a particularly easy and fun way to use yarrow and other recalibrating essences when you are at work.

How Long to Take Flower Essences

The main question I get from people is, "Will I need to take flower essences for the rest of my life?" The answer is no, unless you want to. Since flower essences are not chemical medicines, there are no hard and fast rules. In general, therapy with a flower essence practitioner works like this: The practitioner chooses the most helpful essences for the client. The client uses those essences for about a month. By that time, a healing shift will have occurred such that the client will most likely want to change their essences to address the next "layer" of concern. Of course, there are sometimes essences that a person chooses to take for a longer period of time to continue working on deeper and deeper levels.

In regard to yarrow flower essences, some people like to have it on hand all the time to take again whenever they are stressed or may be attending a very crowded event, for example. Other people work with yarrow for a while, feel the beneficial effects, and then no longer feel the need to use it. Each person's life circumstances and energy are a little different, so the point is that you can use flower essences as a support in the way that works best for you. Some people incorporate flower essences as part of their continual, evolving healing journey, but it's not required.

No Side Effects

People always ask me if flower essences have any side effects. (Like I said, we are indoctrinated to think only of chemical medicines with their myriad of secondary effects.) Most everything you read about flower essences will respond "no." They are energetic remedies, so there are no side effects. But to be comprehensive, I will say that there are really only two things to be aware of in relation to your response to flower essence remedies:

1. Whether you like the preservative: As mentioned above, I've encountered a small amount of clients who really don't care for the alcohol preservative. In those cases, I suggest other brands such as Green Hope Farm, or I instruct the client on how to use the remedies externally instead of internally.

2. The action of emotional clearing: Some flower essences unearth old emotional debris in order to clear it out. This can sometimes be a little startling to people, as it can bring even deeply buried feelings up into conscious awareness. But it really is important for our health to clean out old, buried junk. How can we redefine ourselves and evolve if we are heavy with old emotional hurts or encumbered by limiting beliefs?

Sometimes people find it uncomfortable as these old emotions rise up into conscious awareness. How uncomfortable it is depends upon how much you had accepted that old resentment or belief into your core, and it depends upon how much time you have in your life to do things that aid the clearing, such as exercise, journaling, and generally taking care of yourself.

I'm only telling you this in the spirit of 100 percent truth about the powerful emotional healing that flower essences can provide. This is not to dissuade you in any way from using them. If you ever begin to feel like it is a bit too much, simply take the flower essence remedy less often or take a short break, but then go back to it.

This does not happen with remedies such as yarrow. It only occasionally occurs with remedies that specifically address old resentments, particularly baggage from family issues. You will know if it is that kind of remedy from the description. Here's an example: *Evening primrose from FES assists with healing of painful early emotions such as feeling rejected or unwanted. It especially relates to mother issues.*

Let me explain just a little more as to why it's a beneficial, healing thing to unearth and release these issues. Continuing with the example of evening primrose—if you felt rejected by your mother, it's likely that this is a core issue that pervades your life more than you'd like to admit. It may color all your relationships, making you quick to feel rejected and unwanted. It may have left you unwilling to have your own children. It may have altered your self-esteem, always shadowing you with a feeling of unworthiness.

You could be in counseling for years and never fully release and transcend these issues. You may intellectually understand how it happened or why you have the emotions, but releasing them and changing something so deeply rooted as your own feelings of self-worth are another matter.

Why would it be so intellectually elusive? If you've always felt unwanted by your mother, then you started feeling that way when you were little, long before you could verbalize or intellectually grasp the situation. You began feeling rejected when you were far too young to have any understanding of your mother's life circumstances or the reasons she behaved as she did.

As quantum remedies, flower essences actually can tap into those preintellectual responses, bring them up into our conscious mind so we have new *ah-ha* moments we never had before, and aid us in finally releasing them.

How does this relate to sensitivity? First off, sensitive people have a perpetual struggle with self-worth as it is. We need to do everything we can to reclaim our right to feel confident and okay with who we are.

Secondly, the reason sensitive people often go through life with a general feeling of unease is that we crave clarity, peace, and balance.

When old emotional scars eat away at us, we aren't able to ignore them forever. Our sensitive nature pushes us internally to clear the discordant stuff out, and we will feel uncomfortable (or have more severe symptoms such as depression, anxiety, or ill health) until it is gone.

I am not saying that flower essence therapy is the one and only means to accomplish emotional clearing. There are many healing modalities that may work well for you including hypnotherapy, EFT, pranic healing, regular yoga practice, etc.

It comes down to what is available to you, what you are drawn to, and how much time and resources you have. I recommend flower essences because I do love the yarrows, as they are unique in how they recalibrate sensitivity. But as far as convenience goes, flower essences can be used by anyone without a great deal of effort or time. They are relatively inexpensive, can easily be ordered directly from the manufacturers listed in appendix B, and can be used in ways that easily fit within your own lifestyle. Plus there are options for how to use them.

Evolution of Flower Essence Therapy

Since flower essences are in the category of quantum healing modalities, it may not surprise you that some people are figuring out how to access the flower energy in ever more unique ways.

Both FES and Alaskan Essences have very nice decks of cards with beautiful photographs of the flowers and affirmations or keywords. The cards can be used as a divination deck to help you choose the most beneficial essences for you at this time.

I consider the cards to be a type of flower essence art, and I'm aware of another flower essence practitioner who has taken this art even a step further. At the time of this writing, Ursula Selwood in Ireland is creating very beautiful abstract art based on her flower photos. Just as flower energy can be transferred to water for the remedies, Ursula is successfully experimenting with transferring the flower energy to images that you can view on your computer screen. Why not? Quantum energy doesn't have to follow our rules. (See Appendix B: Flower Essence Resources for information on Ursula's work).

Flower essences are a generous offering from nature to support humanity and help us evolve into the radiant, confident, peaceful beings we are meant to be. They are a special gift to sensitive people, as we are the ones who can best sense their energies and benefit most from the essences' healing vibrations.

· · · · · · · · · · ·

In the next chapter, we'll get a little more grounded again and talk about some of the most exasperating issues sensitive people encounter—physical sensitivities such as chemical and food intolerances.

CHAPTER 6

Stopping Never-Ending Sensitivity Syndrome

In this chapter, we're going to address what a lot of people consider the most vexing irritants about being sensitive, things like food intolerances and chemical sensitivities.

There are plenty of resources out there that teach about the toxicity of our environment—nasty chemicals in our household products, pesticides on our food, chlorine in our water, and mold in the air. It's a never-ending list. Also, there are many dieticians and health practitioners who educate (almost to the point of preaching) about the risks to our internal organs and body functioning. The topics of excessive yeast, heavy metal toxicity, and leaky gut are almost becoming common knowledge, and sensitivity is becoming more and more the norm.

I certainly don't need to repeat any of that in this book, nor do I want to. That would go against the point of this chapter, which is to give you some entirely new ways to reframe your physical sensitivities and begin unraveling them so they are no longer limiting your life excessively.

The following discussion is for adults who are getting frustrated with their multiplying sensitivities (I don't have space in this book to address the considerations for children and babies who are born with obvious sensitivities).

Also please note for the following discussion that I am referring to food *intolerances*, not all-out life-threatening anaphylactic allergic reactions and not celiac disease. Those require additional considerations, but you may find that addressing the psychological and energetic parts of these things can improve even what may seem like permanent diagnoses.

Physical Sensitivity in Adulthood

Common triggers that initiate and perpetuate sensitivities include:

> **Environmental and Chemical Triggers:** Perfumes; fragranced body products and household items; fabric softeners; cleaning products; pesticides; herbicides; the electromagnetic frequencies (EMF) from TVs, computers, microwaves, cell phones, and wireless equipment; fluorescent lights; and mold
>
> **Food Triggers:** Sugar; wheat; corn; dairy; eggs; soy; nuts; additives such as food coloring and monosodium glutamate (MSG)

So in regard to all these myriad of environmental and food irritants... what in the heck is going on? It's as if our bodies are rejecting 80 percent of the world we live in. Or that 80 percent of the world is bad for us, depending upon your perspective.

For sensitive people, these reactions can at times be debilitating. I know this all too well on a personal basis in addition to working with many frustrated, struggling clients. I have traversed through extreme chemical sensitivities such that I could barely walk through a superstore past the laundry and cleaning products aisles. I'd get brain fog, a headache, and nausea just from being in that section of the store. I experienced times when I was massively uncomfortable using my cell phone. I could feel the EMF, and it felt like radioactive poison to my cellular structure. I still feel that way to a certain degree about microwave ovens.

And don't even get me started about food sensitivities. The first item my body rejected was sugar. A donut would make me feel sick and woozy. Then no more gluten, and a cascade through the years such that I ended up with the following diet: no sugar, gluten, soy, eggs, or dairy. I knew things had gone too far when I could barely eat rice, nuts, or even some vegetables. My diet had gone far beyond "clean" to extremely limited and inconvenient. It was neither life sustaining nor healthy at that point. It was hard for me to be happy, and my vitality was very low because I was not getting a sufficient amount of food, no matter how much healthy food I ate.

Never-Ending Sensitivity Syndrome (NESS)

I've witnessed countless sensitive people get caught up in this vicious cycle. I've seen it so often that I've decided it needs its own acronym: NESS or Never-Ending Sensitivity Syndrome. Although I'm going to discuss this primarily in regard to food intolerances, keep in mind that environmental and chemical sensitivities get lumped into this, too.

NESS is the condition in which a sensitive individual continuously develops new or heightened environmental and food sensitives. His well-intentioned healthy diet may begin simply enough by avoiding gluten and maybe one other food group. Then over time, numerous additional intolerances emerge and further restrict the person's diet ... all this *despite* the fact that he is following a physical healing regime prescribed by nutritionists.

Another way NESS manifests is with those who have a food sensitivity that seems to resolve, but then is quickly replaced by a different food. This resembles a never-ending carousel of new symptoms created by new food sensitivities.

How do you know if you are in the throes of NESS? Easy—it has been going on for way too many years. NESS is the ultra-frustrating, seemingly hopeless scenario that occurs after years of trying your best to do everything "right." You've followed the protocols of detoxification, gut healing, and eating fresher, organic, purer foods, and yet intolerance symptoms not only continue but worsen.

I am not speaking to those of you who have been doing the "clean up your diet thing" for only six months. But, it is still useful for you to read this, so that your six months does not turn into fifteen years, as it has for many others.

I also am not particularly addressing those of you whose food reactions are manageable. Let's say you've eliminated gluten from your family's diet and that is working well, with everyone feeling much better. Yet, I encourage you to keep the next part of this discussion in the back of your mind just in case you start down the path of developing even more food sensitivities.

What are the solutions to turn NESS around? You should be able to guess that it obviously doesn't come from the physical-only approach. That method is useful for a while to detoxify our bodies. But remaining only in the physical is a huge part of the problem.

Anti-NESS Tip #1
Food intolerances are only about now *at this moment in time*
For many years the process of cleaning up my diet and healing my gut had seemed quite logical. At the time, I was limiting my foods based on my symptoms. Gluten made me so tired I was incapacitated with fatigue. Dairy resulted in sinus blockage such that I couldn't breathe. Soy led to a cough. Eggs made me nauseous. The formula seemed loud and clear. Particular food = specific problem. My body seemed to be speaking to me clearly about what to eliminate.

What I didn't realize at the time though was just how much our body wisdom lives in the present moment of right now. It was communicating to me what I needed to avoid *at that moment in time*. It meant nothing about the future. To put it another way, my innate wisdom was telling me exactly what I needed to know right then. Period. My mind took that information and over-interpreted it, especially as the passage of time made my mind think it was logical to consider it all as permanent.

The present moment of now is a surprisingly elusive concept for our minds to truly embrace. We automatically have the following thought processes: "Gluten is making me sick. When I don't eat it, I feel better. Well, I guess that's the way it is from now on." *Whoa, whoa, whoa!* The body didn't say that it would be from now on, in perpetuity. As a matter of fact, it is impossible for our innate wisdom to say that. It only knows *now*.

I understand fully how intensely ill we sometimes feel in reaction to certain foods. I've felt those sickening sensations, including incapacitating fatigue, constant constipation and digestive bloating, headaches, nausea, and an overall malaise as if my cells were being ripped apart. I was so ill at times that I didn't want to go on living that way. It was impossible to function.

And that is another reason why it simply makes logical sense to our minds to assume that a dietary reaction is permanent. "Hey, I *never* want to feel that sick again, so no eggs for me." But as a sensitive person, you have the ability to evolve and change.

Anti-NESS Tip #2
Move from the negative to a positive approach full of possibilities

So why is the body telling us to eliminate particular foods in the first place? What's the reason? Is it because the food itself is a toxic poison? Is it because our body needs to detoxify due to overconsumption, or is it because our physical body (and energy body) need to take a break in order to recalibrate and readjust how we process and digest certain foods (or maybe all foods)?

The last one is something we rarely, if ever, consider. It's easy to think of certain foods as "bad." I mean, it's really easy. Overly processed white sugar, gluten in everything, dairy produced in a factory-like, inhumane manner. That's bad, right?

Well, it's certainly not ideal. But what happens, for example, when your body rejects all dairy, even the cheese lovingly handcrafted by a small, locally-sourced company? Food sensitivities are not as simple as good food vs. bad food, and they're not as cut and dried as simply a physical detoxification process.

Food intolerances are becoming so common that there is a lot of education available on the matter. And it always goes like this: *You must heal your gut. Repair your intestinal mucosa by removing all offending foods, do a candida cleanse, use anti-inflammatory herbs and supplements, be sure to take probiotics, etc, etc.* It's a purely physiological perspective that many health practitioners espouse as 100 percent dogma fact. "This is what you *must* do to heal your gut."

I'm not saying there isn't merit to eating healthier and being kinder to our insides, but when well-meaning healing information becomes gospel, the big picture is lost. We no longer see the forest for the trees.

This dogma leads down a never-ending path of discomfort for many sensitive people. They've done all the things suggested to heal their digestive tract, yet their sensitivities and autoimmune reactions of illness only increase. Why? The physiological answer is, "Oh, well, you have leaky gut—an irritated intestinal lining that allows inappropriate molecules into the bloodstream triggering an autoimmune response."

And what is the treatment for leaky gut? Answer: *You must heal your gut. Repair your intestinal mucosa by removing all offending foods, do a candida cleanse, use anti-inflammatory herbs and supplements, be sure to take probiotics, etc and etc.* But didn't I just do all that?!? And so the circle of frustration continues with no apparent end.

Let's start thinking about this from some different perspectives. Consider this: Everything I described above is a blaming, negative kind of approach.

It makes it very easy to fall into the trap that is entirely not helpful for sensitive people—the acceptance that "there is something wrong with me." It perpetuates thoughts such as, "My digestive system is messed up and overly sensitive. I've eaten poorly throughout my life and brought this on." All this unfortunately resonates perfectly with the sensitive person identity we need to transcend, which is: "I am different, my body is overwhelmed, and I cannot tolerate or process the stimuli in this world."

It also falls exactly into the type of thinking I mentioned in chapter 1: "The world outside of me is toxic and too harsh, and I become overwhelmed by it all."

So whether you believe that you are messed up and need to be fixed in order to have a tougher, less-leaky digestive system, or whether you believe that the foods we have available are toxic and bad—both are quite negative, antagonistic ways of conceptualizing it all.

Living in negativity only perpetuates further negativity. Sorry, folks, but that's just the way it works. So consider instead more positive, inclusive possibilities such as, "My body is recalibrating so that I digest my food better than ever. The world is full of nutritious, healthy, vibrant food. Every food has positive qualities and energy my body can use."

Anti-NESS Tip #3
Remember that your digestive system is not isolated all on its own; it is integrated with everything else about you in body, mind, and spirit

When we are frustrated with multiple food intolerances, we should not ignore that our digestive issues and all other aspects of our sensitivity will have common themes running through them. Reread this paragraph from chapter 1 about how we used to always think of ourselves as sensitive people:

"One of the sure signs of a truly sensitive person is that he or she feels animosity toward his or her sensitive nature. Most sensitive people whole-heartedly wish they were tougher and more thick-skinned. They feel like (and have been told) their sensitivity is a weakness. They wish things didn't bother them so much. They wish their emotions weren't so obvious to other people. They wish they could let things go and not worry so much. They aren't comfortable with their sensitivity, and they wish they could do something to get rid of it (or at least get rid of the uncomfortable aspects of it). They are tired of feeling overwhelmed."

Continuing the theme, in chapter 3 I discussed empathic ability. Recall our discussion of how empathic ability feels when it is unbalanced, *"I feel like I am an emotional sponge. I can't handle being around certain people. Sometimes I am overwhelmed with emotions, and I have no idea how to stop them or even where they are coming from. Yet even when I avoid people, I still feel depressed and overly emotional."*

The same symptom-perpetuating themes run through *all* of these scenarios:

1. **Identifying oneself as weak or broken:** "I am overwhelmed with emotion and depressed." "I am too sensitive and not as tough as other people." "My gut doesn't work as it should because I have candida overgrowth and an irritated intestinal lining."

2. **Feeling exposed and trespassed upon:** "I feel like I am an emotional sponge." "I wish I was more thick-skinned." "I have leaky gut, which means food molecules are passing where they should not be in my body."

3. **Accepting a progressively smaller and smaller cut of the world:** "I can't handle being around certain people." "I need to hide my sensitivity from others at work, so I won't go to that event." "I can't eat that because I can't tolerate gluten."

Do you see the themes? What I'm trying to demonstrate to you here is that the symptoms of our gut (and our immune system in general) are not separate from any other part of our functioning. The digestive process is most certainly not separate from our self-image and it is not separate from all our self-limiting beliefs. They are all tied together.

Trying to maintain a separation by looking at our food and environmental intolerances as purely physical symptoms only leads to their continuation. I'll state that another way.

Your digestion can only function in a way that is consistent with these things:

- *Your identity*, that is, what you believe about who you are. This is your self-image, limitations and all.
- *Your world view*, that is, how you feel about other people and about the world in general, negativity and hopelessness included.
- *Your metaphysical/spiritual beliefs*, that is, how expansive do you think you are? Are you just a physical body skin bag filled with salt water that helplessly reacts to toxins in only one way, or are you much more than that?

Think for a moment about where your digestive organs are located deep inside your body. Not only is your digestive system intertwined with everything that you are, it is at the very core of your being. Doesn't it make sense then that your core beliefs and core feelings about yourself are equal to your core physiological processes such as digestion and elimination?

Therefore, to move beyond NESS it is imperative to become aware of those core beliefs and release and change them as you wish for more freedom. Now, please don't think of this as more work, and "Oh no, now I've got broken beliefs!" All I'm saying here is that our physical sensitivities will lessen when we also incorporate emotional and energetic healing into the picture.

If you can, please take an approach of curiosity. Think of it like wandering through a big, old dusty Victorian house where all the original furnishings and knickknacks and stuff of life have been left undisturbed. You would look at some of the stuff reverently. "Wow, that's beautiful!" And you would react to some of the stuff with, "What the heck was that for?" and "I'm glad I don't have to do it that way anymore!"

The goal, if you insist on having one, is to recalibrate and let go of all beliefs that limit your evolution. Ironically, the more you let go of, the bigger you become in body, mind, and spirit. When limitations are removed, you can embrace anything and everything you want about life.

. . . .

Expanding Beyond Limitations
Drawing Exercise

Get a piece of paper and a pencil. This exercise is not about artistic ability. Simple stick figure drawings work just as well as any other representation. Draw yourself in the middle of the page. Think about what you most like about being a sensitive person and draw a representation of that on the picture of yourself. Some common responses to this are, "I like being unique," "I like being an artist," or "I like helping people."

Next think about the one thing that is most frustrating or that is most limiting for you about being a sensitive person. But this time draw that as separate from the picture of you. It can be on the same piece of paper or even on a different piece of paper if you prefer.

After you have drawn what you like and what you don't like, pause and consider this: Can't you have the thing you like about being sensitive without the limiting thing? They don't have to be intertwined. You've already drawn it that way. Now erase or mark out the limiting thing you drew. If you drew it on a separate piece of paper, wad it up and throw it away.

This exercise is a fundamental step in shifting your identity as a sensitive person—embracing what you like about your sensitivity and removing the things that frustrate you most from your identity of who you are.

Flower essences as discussed in the previous chapter are a wonderful support for this kind of recalibration. You also may want to seek out a metaphysical or holistic healing practitioner who can assist you through various methods to access your inner resources and let go of limiting beliefs. Examples might be practitioners who do holistic psychotherapy, Reiki, EFT, craniosacral therapy, yoga therapy, and whatever else calls to you.

Also refer to the next chapter Meditation & Mindfulness. It is when you are in a quiet, meditative state that you can be aware of the discordant feeling of some of your thoughts and beliefs and gain insight as to how to shift them.

. . . .

Positive Deconstruction

Before I close this chapter, I want to talk about one more scenario that leaves many sensitive people nearly incapacitated with environmental and food sensitivities. For this one, we'll use the terms *evolutionary crisis* and *positive deconstruction*.

Many sensitive people wind up going through a period of time in which everything, and I mean everything, seems to fall apart. It often starts with a serious health condition. For me it was being hospitalized with meningoencephalitis. I've seen clients who started this process with a cancer diagnosis, rapidly deteriorating MS, or a herniated disc requiring back surgery, for a few examples.

In an evolutionary crisis scenario, recovery from the health condition does not go smoothly. Further complications usually happen, often involving strong negative reactions to medications or treatments, sudden increased autoimmune symptoms, or further symptoms such as severe digestive shutdown, major depression, or panic attacks.

It's not uncommon during an evolutionary crisis to begin a divorce or lose a job either. By the time sensitive clients come to me in the throes of an evolutionary crisis, they are usually at their wits' end with no energy left at all to fight it or even try to figure out what is going on anymore.

They are typically surprised when I see it all as a good thing, and I don't try to fix individual symptoms. Instead I view the whole experience as "positive deconstruction." I use this term in its purest sense to mean that the person's persona and beliefs about life are being shattered and forcefully deconstructed by life's events. The complete shattering is necessary in order for the person to then reconstruct her identity in a larger, more positive, freeing way.

We've all either known someone or heard stories of those who have had a brush with death, either their own diagnosis or perhaps something like having a baby who died. Although the experience is horrible in some ways, it changed the person such that he no longer worried about small things. He finally realized "what was most important in life," perhaps changed his career to what he always wanted to do, and lived a more meaningful life from that point forward.

The evolutionary crisis is kind of like that, only the struggle can go on much longer with even deeper quantum recalibration happening within the person's thoughts, psyche, and spirit.

It's a bummer that we modern-day humans need a painful event or series of events such as an evolutionary crisis to shock us out of our overly intellectual limitations. Debilitating events and health crises are the way we clean house, clear and recalibrate our psyches, and open up to our souls.

If you suspect you are in the midst of a positive deconstruction, take heart that, as with everything we've been discussing in this book, you aren't doing anything wrong. It is a situation that needs to be accepted for what it is and for the ways it will allow you to shed all that is unnecessary and embrace everything you want about how you want to live your life.

I felt it important to mention this because sensitive people seem to be especially prone to go through the positive deconstruction experience at some point in their lives. That's why I also call it an evolutionary crisis. Sensitive people aren't content to just go through the motions of life. We want to know more and be more than the average Joe. Although your intellectual mind may try to push it away, you feel how your soul yearns to be known by you. There is a lot to who you are. All those parts want to be at the surface, not buried under the mundane so that you can go through life being 1/1000th of who you really are.

So, for many of us, an eruption happens such that all those parts are violently strewn about, and then comes the process of renovation—choosing what to keep and what to get rid of—re-creating and evolving ourselves into highly perceptive, fully alive humans, armed with vitality and love for life.

And so, where am I in terms of this process? In a *much* more comfortable place than I had been for several years. Now I eat whatever I want, but find that I mostly do crave healthy foods. In regard to environmental sensitivities, I consider the ones I have to be my own preferences, rather than limitations. I prefer to avoid all perfumes and fake-scented products. I have an air purifier I use just in case I unintentionally expose myself to a stinky product. I prefer to avoid microwaves. I prefer to avoid this stuff because I feel much better and stronger without them. Period. That is my right and my choice to arrange my environment thusly.

The steps I and my clients take to navigate through NESS and other seeming complications of sensitivity are all about stepping back into your authentic self. Reducing the noise and the toxins and the unbalanced energies is not a limitation at all, but is actually just like parting the curtains to allow the sun to finally enlighten the entire room.

The process is about centering, balancing, developing your sensitive strengths, and claiming your space in the world. I call it the Sensitive (R)evolution.

Part III
Sensitive (R)evolution

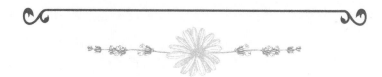

CHAPTER 7

Meditation & Mindfulness

Meditating and learning how to be totally present in the moment of now is important to your recalibration and evolution. Everyone seems to inherently understand the potential benefits of meditation. Yet, I swear, everyone has this same response to the idea of meditation as soon as I bring it up, "Oh, I can't meditate. I don't know how to turn off my mind." I only have this response, "Great! Then you are starting out the same way the world's deepest meditators did."

Meditation does not immediately come easily to anyone. We all have to overcome the following hurdles:

- We were taught to only focus our attention on our thoughts.
- We were never taught that there was any other way to gather information from within ourselves besides thinking.
- Our society puts a lot of pressure on us to constantly think about the future, and when our thoughts wander, they tend to go to regrets of the past and worries about the future.

This is the foundation we're all given in this society, so cut yourself some slack, okay? Given our starting point, how can you possibly expect that you would be able to just plop down one day and calm and clear your mind into a state of blissful oneness with all that is?

First, we need some guidance about how to even start. I like this quote from Jeff Foster: "What is true mediation? Being awake and alive to this precious moment."[13] The goal of meditation isn't to *do* anything. Instead it is simply about being present right here, right now.

And as simple as that is, it absolutely blows our minds. "What?!? I don't have to do anything? How can I do something like meditating, if I'm not doing anything?" And my answer is, "Exactly."

· ·

A Twenty-Day, Four-Step Plan to Change Habits for Mindfulness

Since people get frustrated and tend to give up on meditation, I'm going to present it in a very different way than you might expect. We are not going to jump in to doing meditations. First, I'm going to present you with simple assignments that will build on each other, ultimately making it much easier for you to find some stillness to meditate and also listen to your intuition, which we'll talk more about in chapter 8.

Why do I even have this chapter on meditation in a book about sensitivity? Meditation, which we'll define as "being fully present in the now," is imperative for your sensitive recalibration and evolution by helping you step outside your normal mode of thinking. Thinking got you to exactly where you are today. Thinking will not take you anywhere else other than where you currently are.

In this book, I've mentioned the importance of accepting a new definition of yourself, letting go of limiting beliefs, and listening to your innate wisdom. How do you accomplish those things? Well, you don't. We cannot "accomplish" nor "do" such

---

13. Debra Anderson, "Simple 30-minute Mindful Meditation: An Effortless Receptivity of Life," accessed September 4, 2015, http://www.bodyandsoul.cc/simple -30-minute-mindful-meditation-an-effortless-receptivity-of-life-jeff-foster/.

things, rather we have to slow down a bit and open the door to allow them to unfold.

That kind of evolution will naturally occur once you begin to change the habits of how you normally think. Without really "trying" you will find that one day you suddenly are "in the present moment of now." Even if it starts with only twenty seconds, that is perfect. *Healing evolution happens in between the times when we are thinking as usual.*

Whatever stereotypes you have in your mind about meditation, you don't have to do it that way. Although it's nice to be alone in a quiet room, it isn't always required. You don't have to sit in Lotus pose and chant *om*, although that works too. You can be walking. You can be sitting. You can have silence, or you can listen to a guided meditation. There are many options. Don't worry about that stuff at all yet, or ever. First, we're going to start with practice exercises that will reset the way your brain constantly goes a mile a minute. The first step is changing habits.

Thinking constantly, having our minds going a mile a minute all the time, and being surrounded by constant noise is a habit. Many of you reading this may already have figured out that you prefer regular quiet time to decompress. But there are also lots of you who have to go along with all the noise of the family and the workplace. You're used to constant noise, and you don't consider that it could be any other way. Constant music, radio, and background noise are the habits of our society. That may seem innocuous, but it is not.

The constant thoughts and nonstop noise are a barrier to noticing what is happening in the here and now. The noise makes it quite difficult to be able to hear that still small voice of intuition.

I'm far from the first teacher to say such things. As a matter of fact, here is a quote from Fred Rogers of *Mister Rogers' Neighborhood*: "If we take time, we can often go much deeper

as far as a spiritual life is concerned than we can if there's constant distraction. Often television gives such constant distraction—noise and fast-paced things—which doesn't allow us to
take time to explore the deeper levels of who we are, and who
we can become."[14]

So here is your first "Learn to Be in the Now" assignment:

Assignment #1: Eliminate Extraneous Noise and Be In the Moment

For one week pay attention to only what you are doing in any
given moment. For example, that means no radio or music of
any kind in the car while you're driving. Try not to daydream too
much either because that is "thought" noise. Really pay attention
to the other cars on the road, their colors, and license plates. Pay
attention to the feel of the road and the sounds of your car. Notice some things along the way that maybe you've never paid attention to.

This also means no music or television playing in the background at home while you're making dinner. Just pay close attention to what you're doing. If you are eating, only eat, no
reading at the same time. If you are cleaning up around your
house, only do that, and focus on it as much as you can without thinking about other things.

This one might be a hurdle for some of you—no music in
the ears while running or exercising at the gym. Just as the instructions for driving, simply pay attention to everything around
you and feel the breeze against your skin as you run. It's okay if
you want to give your mind something to focus on; experiment
with mantras or affirmations while you are not listening to music. This would be something like repeating in your mind, "I am
lighter and stronger with each step." But also try thinking about

14. Amy Hollingsworth, *The Simple Faith of Mister Rogers: Spiritual Insights from the World's Most Beloved Neighbor* (Nashville, TN: Thomas Nelson, 2007), 3.

absolutely nothing and only noticing what is happening in each moment.

If you go to the gym and background music or a TV is playing that you cannot control, don't worry about it. Simply continue the pattern of paying attention to what you are doing, feeling, and experiencing in each moment. Notice the texture and feel of the barbells and the refreshing feel of the water when you take a drink.

Of course all sorts of distracting thoughts will enter your mind as you practice this assignment. No big deal. Just notice the thoughts and let them pass on through.

I also understand that if you have young children, this will be a very different kind of exercise. Do what you can, and try to get some extra time by yourself to have some variety of environments for this assignment. If you have a partner or roommates who have to have the TV on constantly, here's news for them! No, they do not have to have noise constantly. Noise is not a "have to have" situation. It is a habit.

Tell them you are doing this practice exercise and why it's important to you. It is only for one week. Invite them to join you. If they refuse, they can go watch TV elsewhere for the week. And when I say one week for this assignment, I do mean seven days.

For clarity, I don't mean you need to have silence 24/7 for seven days. That's impossible, and not the point anyway. The purpose isn't the elimination of the noise per se, the point is to give your mind space to focus 100 percent on whatever it is you are doing right at that moment. If there is the buzz of background noise, especially talk radio or TV, your mind cannot be 100 percent attentive to whatever you are doing in the present moment. Being focused in this way on what you are doing in the present moment is traditionally called "mindfulness."

Assignment #2: Keep Track of Negative Thoughts

Assignment #1 is about giving your mind some "breathing room" as it were to simplify and focus solely on the now, thus allowing it to stop the pattern of always pushing and rushing ahead. After you've done the first assignment, it will be easier to do this second one, which is to pay attention to what the content of your thoughts actually are.

Let me begin by giving you a little background for the importance of this. I highly recommend the book *The Hidden Messages in Water* by Masaru Emoto. The author is a scientist who developed a method to photograph the crystalline structure of water. The book is filled with beautiful photographs of water crystals. Emoto demonstrated with his real-time photography process that thoughts and intentions directly affected the shape and cohesiveness of the water's crystalline structure.

"Love" and other positive words, such as "cooperation," were shown or said to the water, which was then photographed. The results showed very well-structured, beautiful crystals. Negative phrases like "I hate you," resulted in malformed, loose crystals or no discernible crystalline structure at all. He proved that water was empathic to the max. It directly reflected the energy sent to it, and Emoto demonstrated this in a visual, scientific way.

I recommend you look at the book to see the photos and get the full impact of how the water looked as it reacted to the intent of the energy/thoughts sent to it. So Emoto's work leads to the next logical thought, which is ... human beings are made of a lot of water, right? According to USGS Water Science School, "A human being's brain and heart are composed of 73 percent water and the lungs are about 83 percent water. The skin contains 64 percent water, muscles and kidneys are 79 percent, and even the bones are watery: 31 percent." We are made primarily of water.[15]

---

15. The USGS Water Science School, "The Water in You," accessed July 15, 2015, http://water.usgs.gov/edu/propertyyou.html.

Emoto's photos were clear. Negative words and thoughts destroyed the crystalline structure of the water in his experiments. Now consider this: each and every single thought that flits through your brain affects the crystalline structure of the water in your body. Each and every thought has an impact.

So when you think things like, "I'm so stupid, I never learn," "I hate it when he does that," or you spend time thinking about how angry you are about a particular politician's statements, you have just broken apart the crystalline structure of all the water in your body.

That's just one reason of a thousand why it's beneficial to reel in the negative thoughts. Most people truly have no idea how often they are thinking critical, negative, and unnecessarily harsh thoughts.

So for Assignment #2, get yourself a little notebook or pad of paper and make a tally mark every single time you think a negative or harsh thought. Yes, this exercise is similar to the one we did in chapter 4, but it is different. Chapter 4's exercise was specifically about your own self-defeating thoughts. This exercise is about every negative sort of thought in general. Even if you are a generally positive person, I believe you will be surprised at how often you think things like "I'm so stupid" in response to a simple mistake, "Whoa! I look like crap" when looking in the mirror first thing in the morning, or "Grrr, I'd like to strangle that guy" in response to a news story.

This assignment is only for one full day. All day and up through bedtime, have your notepad with you (or if you know how to do this on your phone, that's fine too) and keep count of every single time a negative or harsh thought crosses your mind, even if fleeting, and even if you think, "Oh, that's just a little thing I say to myself. It doesn't mean anything." Sorry, but to your body, to your psyche, and to your energetic self, every single little thought *does* mean something. It means exactly what it is. If you think, "Oh, I'm so stupid," then you just pronounced, like a mantra or affirmation, that you are stupid. Your body and your energy react accordingly.

So how does this relate to meditation? Remember we defined meditation as being fully present in the moment right now. It's implied that your time in the present moment needs to be at least neutral if not positive for there to be any benefit to turning your attention there.

Also, all those little negative thoughts add up to what? Nothing but noise, completely unnecessary, unhelpful, damaging in fact, noise and static that clogs our minds and prevents us from hearing our body's wisdom clearly.

Though you may not have imagined this was the type of assignment I'd be giving you to learn how to meditate, it is honestly one of the most important exercises you'll ever do. That quiet, peaceful space in your mind does not just happen automatically, you have to reclaim it. And you reclaim it by taking notice of unhelpful habits and making those previously unconscious habits conscious, so that you can then change them.

Assignment #3: Turn Off the News

Assignment #3 may seem similar to #1, which was eliminating all excess noise, but this one is much more specific. Do this one for at least five days at a separate time after you have done assignments #1 and #2. "News" programs, whether they are on television, radio, or the sensationalized videos we click online, are a special, particularly inflammatory type of "noise." They distract us from the present moment by inciting our base emotional responses of fear and anger, causing a flood of unnecessary, agitating thoughts.

Your response to this may be, "Five days with no news?!? I'll be misinformed. I won't know what's going on in the world." Uh, take it easy. If anything really important or interesting happens, you can be sure a friend or a family member will tell you. Anything that isn't really important, well, it really isn't important, is it? You won't have wasted your time and energy listening and thinking about it.

This assignment also applies to social media and links in e-mails, etc. For five days, do not click on anything that is going to lead to disturbing, misleading, or highly charged "news." Don't tell me you don't know what it is until you click. It's pretty easy to tell, my perceptive, sensitive friend. If in doubt, err on the side of not clicking.

The reasons for doing this exercise are multifold. Most news stories are upsetting in nature. You are a sensitive person. Nothing good comes from willingly allowing yourself to be agitated on a regular basis. It is distracting and separates you yet again from that centered, focused place in your mind. This exercise will clarify how that is manifesting in your life. Then you can choose how and where to obtain the news that will be best for your peace of mind, rather than just doing it because it seems like everyone "should" watch the news.

Assignment #4: Daily Mindfulness for Seven Days

In assignment #1 we broached the concept of "mindfulness." Now it's time to participate more fully in mindfulness exercises. Mindfulness is ridiculously helpful for sensitive people, so that is why I am specifically calling it out in our meditation chapter. It's a practice that is so in tune with sensitivity it is as if it was designed just for us highly perceptive people. Practicing mindfulness teaches us to eliminate the constant static and noise in our minds. It sharpens our focus, expands our intuition and awareness, and gives us a platform to fully use and finally appreciate our highly perceptive senses. It is a key ingredient to sensitive evolution.

So your one-week mindfulness assignment is to do at least one mindfulness exercise per day for seven days straight. Another part of the beauty of mindfulness practice is that it merges right into whatever you are already doing, no need to set any time aside. Following are seven mindfulness exercises to get you started.

Day 1—Mindful Eating

This time-honored eating mindfully exercise is from Dr. Jon Kabat-Zinn,[16] who popularized Mindfulness Based Stress Reduction in the 1980s. This practice is based on ancient Buddhist teaching. If you don't like raisins, just use any other food.

1. Sit comfortably in a chair.
2. Place a raisin in your hand.
3. Examine the raisin as if you had never seen it before.
4. Imagine it as its "plump self" growing on the vine surrounded by nature.
5. As you look at the raisin, become conscious of what you see: the shape, texture, color, and size. Is it hard or soft?
6. Bring the raisin to your nose and smell it.
7. Are you anticipating eating the raisin? Is it difficult not to just pop it in your mouth?
8. How does the raisin feel? How small is it in your hand?
9. Place the raisin in your mouth. Become aware of what your tongue is doing.
10. Bite ever so lightly into the raisin. Feel its squishiness.
11. Chew three times and then stop.
12. Describe the flavor of the raisin. What is the texture?
13. As you complete chewing, swallow the raisin.
14. Sit quietly, breathing, aware of what you are sensing.

Dr. Kabat-Zinn describes this type of mindfulness exercise, saying, "The raisin exercise dispels all previous concepts we may be harboring about meditation. It immediately places it in the realm of the ordinary, the everyday, the world you already

---

16. Mark Williams, John Teasdale, Zindel Segal, and Jon Kabat-Zinn, *The Mindful Way Through Depression: Freeing Yourself from Chronic Unhappiness* (New York: Guilford Press, 2007), 55.

know but are now going to know differently. Eating one raisin very, very slowly allows you to drop right into the knowing in ways that are effortless, totally natural, and entirely beyond words and thinking. Such an exercise delivers wakefulness immediately. There is in this moment only tasting." [17]

Day 2—Mindful Walking [18]

Start with only five or ten minutes of mindful walking time. That is actually more than it seems. If you want to take a longer walk, do ten minutes of mindful walking first, then continue to walk as you choose after that.

For this mindful walk, focus on only one of your senses at a time. Think of that sense as the anchor for your attention. Focus on the physical feeling of your gait as your feet hit the ground. For another walk, focus on the sounds that come and go as you move through your environment. Continue to bring your attention back to that sense over and over whenever thoughts or reactions arise.

Day 3—Mindful Listening [19]

This exercise is designed to open your ears to sound in a completely accepting way. So much of what we see and hear on a daily basis is influenced by thoughts of past experiences. Mindful listening helps us leave the past where it is and come into a neutral, present awareness.

Select a new piece of music from your music collection, something you've never heard before but makes you wonder what it might sound like. It's also okay to choose something you haven't listened to for a very long time. Close your eyes and use

---

17. Dr. Freddy Jackson Brown, *Get the Life You Want: Finding Meaning and Purpose through Acceptance and Commitment Therapy* (London, England: Watkins, 2013), 140–141.
18. Kate Sciandra, *The Mindfulness Habit: Six Weeks to Creating the Habit of Being Present* (Woodbury, MN: Llewellyn Publications, 2015), 120.
19. Alfred James, "6 Mindfulness Exercises You Can Try Today," accessed July 11, 2015, http://www.pocketmindfulness.com/6-mindfulness-exercises-you-can-try-today/.

headphones if you can. Don't think about the genre or the artist. Instead, allow yourself to get lost in the journey of sound for the duration of the song. Allow yourself to explore the intricacies of the music. Let your awareness climb inside the track and play among the sound waves.

The idea is to just listen and allow yourself to become fully entwined with what is being played/sung, without preconception or judgment of the genre, artist, lyrics, instrumentation, or its origin.

Day 4—Mindful Object Acknowledgment

This exercise is to look at something that you normally take for granted in a new way. Choose something in your environment that has been sitting there untouched for a long time. If you are inside, a good choice is a knickknack on the shelf. Pick up the item and notice the following things: How heavy is it? Close your eyes and feel its texture and shape in your fingers. Now open your eyes and look closely at the intricacies of how it was made. Where was it made? Give it a gentle cleaning if it needs dusting from sitting on the shelf for a while. Then put it back or display it in a new place.

Day 5—Mindful Mundane Chore

Choose a simple task like washing the dishes or sweeping the floor. This should be a task in which you normally would go on autopilot and your mind would wander. In this instance, approach the task differently and only pay close attention to what you are doing. If you are sweeping, notice the feel of the handle in your hand; listen to sound of the bristles as they touch the floor. If thoughts do intrude, just let them drift by, and return your attention to your activity.

Day 6—Mindful Olfactory Sense

Smell something with a natural scent that you really like. It may be your cup of coffee or tea, an orange, a flower in your yard, or a whiff from a bottle of essential oil. Pay close attention to what happens in your nose as you inhale the scent. How long does the scent linger and where do you notice it? What happens to your breathing when you inhale the scent? How does it make you feel?

Day 7—Mindful Shower

The shower is another place we normally allow our thoughts to meander. In this shower exercise, start your mindfulness from the moment you touch the faucet. Notice the feel and temperature of the faucet as you turn it on. Then pause and listen to the sound of the water as it hits the different surfaces. It will sound different when it hits the shower curtain vs. the tub or your skin. Feel the temperature of the water and how deeply you can sense that within your skin. When thoughts arise, just return your attention to the shower. Notice how the humid air feels in your nose as you inhale. Then when you are done showering, continue to notice the nuances of how the towel feels against your skin as you dry.

Once you have gone through your seven-day assignment, it will start to feel natural to make mindfulness a part of your day-to-day life. I can't overstate the importance of actually doing all these assignments in order and dedicating the time to each one for a total of twenty days.

1. Eliminate extraneous noise for one week and pay attention to what you are doing in that moment—7 days
2. Keep track of negative thoughts—1 day
3. Turn off the news—5 days
4. Daily mindfulness—7 days

Once you have done this series of progressive exercises for the twenty days, then you can consider doing what you probably thought I'd begin with in this chapter, listening to guided meditations. Your mindfulness practice will help you tremendously when it comes time to slow down and focus your attention within for meditation. Mindfulness teaches you to reconnect with your senses and fully engage in your experiences. This skill transfers perfectly to meditation. The following guided meditation is training and practice for doing just that—engaging all your senses into your meditation experience.

. . . .

Using All Five Senses
Beach Relaxation Meditation

Sit comfortably with your back supported and your feet flat on the floor. Shift or move so you are very comfortable. Adjust your clothing if needed. Take in a relaxing breath and slowly exhale. Now imagine yourself at a peaceful, beautiful ocean beach. This may be a beach you've been to before, or it may be your ideal fantasy beach. In either case, the setting is perfect. The weather is exactly as you like it. You have everything you need...

Begin by looking around and really noticing what your beach looks like. How many clouds are in the sky? What color is the sand? What color is the water, and how does it change as you look farther out? Look down at yourself and notice what you are wearing. Let your eyes relax as you gaze far, far off in the distance where you can see a couple tiny ships. You wonder how far away they must be. You can see the gentle curve of the horizon...

Listen and notice what sounds you hear at your beach. Tune in to the ebb and flow of the waves. Notice what other sounds you hear. You may hear the call of a seagull. The ocean breeze makes a subtle sound as it gently blows by your ears. Notice what other sounds you hear...

Take in a deep breath through your nose and notice the ocean air... How does it smell? You may notice other smells at your beach too like the smell of your suntan lotion.

Now you notice some seashells near you. Pick one up. What does it feel like in your hand? Is it smooth or rough or some of both? Stop and notice the warmth of the sun on your skin and how that feels ... How does the sand feel beneath your feet? Feel free to step into the waves and notice how the water feels. What temperature is it? How does it feel against your skin?

Also notice how you are feeling in this place. Are you relaxed? Happy? How do the energies of this beautiful, natural place affect you?

Now walk back to your towel or beach chair where you will find a refreshing beverage waiting for you. It is your favorite drink. Pick it up and take a drink, noticing the taste. Is it simple? Or is it complex with different flavors? Take one more sip and enjoy all the sights, sounds, and feelings of your perfect beach ... Know that you can come back to this place anytime you want.

Return your attention back to your body sitting in the chair. Hear the sounds in the room around you. Wiggle your fingers and toes ... take in a nice, deep, energizing breath, and when you are ready, open your eyes.

· · · · · · · · · · ·

You can look to Appendix C: Guided Meditations for Sensitive People for more meditations that are particularly useful for grounding, calming, and clearing. Your new skills in mindfulness and meditation will help you tremendously to focus your attention inward and learn more about your intuition and empathic sensitivity. For more about that, let's move on to the next chapter.

CHAPTER 8

Making Friends with Your Intuition & Empathic Ability

We've established throughout this book that sensitive, highly perceptive people naturally have strong intuition. Yet why does intuition seem so elusive and difficult to understand? Well, one complication is that we're taught our entire lives to dismiss intuition. There is an overwhelming amount of social pressure that we *must* have observable, fact-based reasoning to back up any and all actions we take in this life. Going on a hunch or doing something just because it "feels" right is not only severely frowned upon, but often outright mocked. This is the framework we grow up in from early childhood on! So if you say that you don't know how to be aware of your intuition, much less listen to it for decisions in your life, well, join the club! Most of us are all starting from the same gate of over-intellectualization. The good news, though, is that it is *never* too late to shift gears.

There are quite a few of you reading this book who have already done a lot of work to understand your intuition and empathic senses. You may even be a psychic reader or an intuitive in a professional way. This chapter is still for you. We all experience the frustration of how easy it can be to relate quantum information to our clients, but it is sometimes a whole different ball game when we need that intuitive information for ourselves in our own personal quandaries.

Some of us may feel like we're quite comfortable having one foot in the metaphysical energies all the time. But I know full well that no matter how practiced we may be, we all have times when we misinterpret a feeling or a bit of guidance. Occasionally we'll experience a full on, "Well, I don't know what that was about!" when we are baffled by what the intuitive information was trying to convey or the resulting turn of events.

No matter how comfortable we may become with living by our intuition and metaphysical senses, it still will never be the intellect's native land and will always have an air of mystery and occasional confusion.

The Foreign Country of Intuition

Hopefully you noticed that I named this chapter "Making Friends with Your Intuition & Empathic Ability." I'm phrasing it that way for a few reasons. One is because we start off as strangers to our intuition *and* our minds are prone to misinterpreting the language of intuition. Intuition and empathic ability speak a quantum language. The intellectual thoughts in our brain seriously do not. Beginning to listen to our intuition is a little like our brains going on an unplanned, extended vacation to a surprise foreign country that it didn't have any familiarity with at all.

To take the metaphor further, listening to intuition and empathic, psychic information is like your intellectual thoughts just got parachuted down into the country of Lesotho. Lesotho? You may have never heard of that country ... much less have any knowledge of the language, the customs, the food, or how to get around.

And that, my friends, is exactly what it is like to take those first steps to venture into the metaphysical realm of intuitive and empathic guidance. So be patient with yourself, and recognize that you're embarking on a lifelong journey that will always be a curiosity to your intellect.

Please note: For the initial part of this discussion, I am lumping intuition and empathic ability together as they have many similarities.

Living Intuitively

I originally thought this chapter would be about intuition and empathic development in a more standard way. But it occurred to me that there are already many great books that teach those things, several of which are listed in my resources section. Many skilled teachers and sources are already available for you to learn more about awakening and developing your intuitive resources. Although I will be giving you some tips to get started, I don't want to repeat information when I can, instead, give you something different and not available elsewhere. So what's going to follow in this chapter is vital information that you would likely not be able to easily find from other sources. I want to help you, as a sensitive, highly aware person to navigate your path down the road of living intuitively.

I can't make the road completely smooth and bump-free for you, but this chapter should at least give you a metaphorical pair of binoculars so you can see what is coming up ahead. It will make your journey a little easier and even more fun. Hiccups can happen along the way as you practice incorporating intuition into your daily life. My aim is to help you identify the causes of the most common hurdles and, perhaps, intercept some of the frustrations altogether. Again, that is why I call this chapter "Making Friends." We'll start with a discussion of intuition and then cover empathic ability later.

So you may ask, "What hiccups or frustrations are you talking about? Following my intuition should make my life easier, right?" Sorry, but that is intellectual assumption number one. You just used the judgmental terms "should" and "easier." And so the trouble can sometimes begin ...

There is an important reason I began this chapter with the metaphor of Lethoso. I didn't randomly choose that country. It is a small, somewhat hidden country within the country of South Africa. It's pretty obscure and not understood nor studied by most of the population of earth ... a lot like intuition. In fact, it has so much in common with intuition and our metaphysical sensitivities, that I am going to continue on for a bit.

Here is more information about the country: It is also known as "The Kingdom in the Sky" because of its high elevation. Lethoso is crisscrossed by a network of rivers and mountain ranges. It is home to an incredible amount of poverty, yet it contains some of the most striking and beautiful scenery in the world.

Our intuition is a high vibration kingdom, if you would, land-locked by our intellectual thoughts. It definitely leads us to some of the most striking and beautiful experiences possible in life. But wait, how does poverty fit into the metaphor? All of the "good luck" and wonderfulness of intuition occurs only outside of our materialistic, goal-oriented approach to life. Sorry to go on and on about it, but the metaphor of Lethoso will be easy for you to remember later when you need it … and you will.

Now a story demonstrating exactly how intuition can sometimes go "wrong" when we make it impossible for it to work in any other way. The good news is this story is about kitties and a bunny. Oh, and please feel free to laugh at my mishaps in this tale. I call this: *The Bunny Debacle.*

This story starts with my cat named Merlin. He is a handsome, domestic shorthair kitty with all black fur. He's a good, sweet boy, but as the story began he seemed lonely and bored, so I felt like I should get him a friend. And when I say I "felt" like I should get him a friend, it was my intuition speaking. It wasn't actually my desire. Merlin was easy to take care of, and I had a really peaceful, mellow home. Getting another pet wasn't the "smart" thing to do in my intellectual opinion, but my intuition was nagging me.

We had gotten Merlin from Craigslist a couple years earlier. That had gone really well, so I started looking again on Craigslist for another pet. In my mind, I absolutely did not want to get another cat, though. In my adult life, I had lived with pairs of cats, and the cats never got along. They would often have fights, and it absolutely drove me nuts. I did not want to have that happen again.

So, if not a cat, then what? Dogs were allowed at my apartment, but I knew I didn't have enough space. I got no intuitive hit on that. So no dog. Then one evening I felt the strongest intuitive urge to look on Craigslist again. I clicked on the pets section, and there was an ad for "the most adorable bunny." A bunny rabbit? Really? My intuition said, "Oh, yes, Merlin and the bunny won't fight, and they will play together. It will be cute."

Fast-forward to a couple days later—my daughter and I came home with a dwarf angora bunny rabbit. It was a big puff of fur. It was true that Merlin did not get upset about it. He was mostly curious, and they did even play a bit that evening. It was quite cute. I quickly learned some things I didn't like about how high maintenance a long-furred bunny like that was going to be. *But my intuition had steered me in this direction,* I thought. *So I guess I'll see what happens.* And this is what happened—

That night I woke up with a fever. Intense chills alternating with being drenched in sweat didn't seem like a good sign. By the time I woke up in the morning, my symptoms had worsened to difficulty breathing, shaking, and feeling dizzy. The bunny was killing me! It had to go ASAP! As the morning went on, I got so sick, that I had no qualms about texting the lady to return the bunny *now*. Of course, she was annoyed with me, but I felt like I was going to pass out any moment. It was the bunny or me at that point, and so the bunny went back. I came back home and cleaned and cleaned to get every speck of bunny allergen out of my home.

While I was doing that, my mind was racing, of course. Besides feeling like death warmed over, I felt foolish, embarrassed, and definitely had a whole lot of, "What in the heck was that about?" going on. The intuitive urge to get the bunny had seemed so strong and clear. Yet, the results appeared disastrous.

I was so ill it only would have been worse if I had wound up in the hospital, which I nearly did. I inconvenienced people, disappointed my daughter, and wasted a lot of time. Those close to me know that I live very much by my intuition, so what was I going to tell them? I didn't want to demonstrate a terrible intuition example. So that's the state of mind where I was for a while.

Later that day, I needed to return the bunny items I had purchased. My daughter and I were at a pet store doing a return when we noticed that there was an adorable litter of little black kittens available for adoption. *Sigh.* Can you see where this story is going? Well, at that moment in time I was still knee deep in "What happened? Did I misinterpret something?" to totally get it yet, although I had an inkling.

We observed the kittens, and the littlest one, a female with a light pink collar, seemed different from the rest of the litter. She was off to the side playing by herself. She looked up and made serious eye contact with me, unlike any of the other kittens. We asked to meet her, and she was sweet as could be, letting us hold her for a long time while purring. I felt guilty about putting my daughter through the bunny ordeal, and that left me much more inclined than I ever would have been to say, "Okay, kitten instead."

It was finally beginning to dawn on me that I had put myself through the wringer all because of my absolute refusal to even consider a kitty in the first place, plus I had engaged in some other serious anti-intuition mind-sets.

The conclusion of the story: Hermione (my daughter chose the kitten's name) is a truly adorable, smart, sweet cat. Merlin had some normal feline issues adapting to her arrival, but they were pretty mild, and our home is harmonious. I am very glad we adopted Hermione. I love her energy, and I believe she will continue to do a lot to teach me about living in harmony with my intuition.

How do I know it was intuition leading me to the little kitten? Wasn't it just giving in after screwing up?

Well no, I certainly didn't need to give in. I had good physical reasons for returning the bunny, and my daughter actually was not that broken up about it because she said she was having allergic symptoms too. I could have easily maintained my "no cat" stance if I wanted.

I have used my intuition enough in my life that I can tell full well when I am getting an intuitive feeling vs. having an intellectual idea, goal, or thought. They feel different in my body. A thought feels like it's happening up in my head between my ears. Plus a thought is usually in response to some association or train of thought I have started. An intuitive feeling has a different quality, and I sense it down in my body. Sometimes intuitive feelings just pop up unexpectedly. The bunny debacle was instigated by an intuitive feeling. I knew that 100 percent, so what went wrong?

Upon reflection, it was easy for me to realize that the way I had been approaching the pet issue, I *never* would have been in that particular pet store, especially at that time, except that I was absolutely intent that I had to return the bunny stuff. I also *never* would have considered adopting from the rescue at the pet store. I preferred to look on Craigslist for a lower cost or free pet. I realized that I had just gone on a very bumpy, uncomfortable journey to get myself in the right place at the right time to find our next ideal pet. Intuition does not have to work this way! It would far prefer to take the enjoyable path of least resistance at all times.

So why was the path to little Hermione so incredibly convoluted and painful? Because I had every major barrier to intuition up and running: *resistance, judgment,* and *fear.*

These three things are indeed poison to the flow of intuitive information. I limited my options based on past experiences. I had narrowed the potentials for what I would even allow the outcome to be. I also closed off the means by which I was willing to listen. And I was being swayed by fear, the most deadly barrier of all to the intuitive process. Let's review each of these.

Resistance

I was dead set against getting a cat. That pretty much sums that one up. Before even getting started, I had closed off the direct route to the kitten. The intuitive detour signs were up immediately. Intuition and synchronicity could only work around the barrier I had already erected.

Judgment

I was operating from the purview (pun intended) of judgment. That is, my intellect had formed a conclusion from past "evidence" that two cats would never get along.

Remember I said that in my adult life I had only personally known cats that fought a lot. My mind took that to a forgone conclusion (i.e., that was all I had known, so that was the only way it ever could be).

The moment I realized that my own intellectual barriers had waylaid intuition's route, it became completely obvious to me that of course, there are many cats in the world who live together and get along.

When I actually stopped and reconsidered my thoughts about it, I realized that it was the way we had introduced the cats in our past that caused the lousy relationships.

Isn't it silly how that possibility didn't even occur to me until I had gone through this entire ordeal? But that is how entrenched beliefs become, and how shaken up we have to be before we'll reconsider those beliefs.

Our intellect is very proud of how it learns from past experience. It files those memories away and always brings it all up again with any similar situation saying something like, "Oh no, you've seen this before and it never works out. Remember this and this and this." That part of our intellect records history—the actions and the results—and that's all it does. It doesn't occur to it to think outside the box and say, "Well, that outcome happened in the past. Let's figure out a better way." Allowing for a truly different way, and an outcome never before seen—that's not the way of the intellect, rather it's the domain of intuitive, quantum thought.

Fear

And why was I so dead set against a cat? Because I was *afraid* they would fight, based on my past negative experiences. Fear is the most typical emotional blockade to intuition and synchronicity, which prevents us from seeing through to the clear and easy path.

I also had money-based fear. That's a big one for many of us. I didn't want to spend the money on a kitten because my income had been less lately, and it seemed to me like an irresponsible way to direct my funds in my given situation. Never mind that I had just had a healing session the previous week that addressed exactly that. *Whew*, the fear and judgment based approach to money is very much the way of our world, and, to be honest, I am still figuring how to step out of it entirely.

Limiting your intuitive possibilities due to worrying about the money you think is or will be available is *always* based in fear. What will people think? How will I pay this other bill later? And so you might ask, "But isn't that just being responsible?"

Intuition does not buddy up to the concept of responsibility. Being "responsible" is a judgment. It's an intellectual limitation that blocks what intuition and synchronicity can bring to you. And no, I'm not giving you the go ahead to spend all your money like a maniac. What I am saying is this: Be clear about what you feel is coming (a new pet, a new job, a new place to live, a fun vacation) then *do not* limit what you think is possible based on the monetary funds currently available.

If you allow intuition and synchronicity to guide you down the smooth, easy path to the best outcome, then things will happen that you hadn't considered, such as the tax refund arrives that you had forgotten about or a friend suddenly invites you to join her on a low-cost fun trip to your dream destination. The point is *you don't know what you don't know, but intuition does.*

Here is one more very important lesson about following your intuition: *Don't assume that the start is the finish.* There are several reasons why intuition may have to lead us through a circuitous route. In the bunny debacle story, it was my intellectual barriers that made me have to take the long, hard road to a kitten. It would have been a bummer if I had assumed, "Well, I was wrong," and stopped listening at that point. I would have been left with nothing but confusion.

Also please keep in mind that our desires also intersect with other people's lives. Obtaining a new job or purchasing your perfect home requires those people on the other end to leave their job to create a vacancy for you, or to decide one day to put their house on the market. You may get a strong intuitive feeling about something, but a bit of time may need to pass for the rest of the people involved in the big picture to get their affairs in order so synchronicity can then jump in.

So this is another situation where you might worry that you heard your intuition incorrectly. Our own impatience can create a complicated route when we assume that what we see in the beginning of the intuitive process is the final outcome. Don't let impatience make you give up on an intuitive feeling.

Remember chapter 6 about evolutionary crisis and positive deconstruction? The point of the deconstruction is to "take the blinders off." The crisis dismantles things like your limiting beliefs, your over-intellectualization of all that is, and your stubborn insistence upon forcing what you *think* is best rather than allowing what is divinely wonderful.

So, in the end, the outcome of the evolutionary crisis is a good one, and you will be surprised at the ease and simplicity intuition can take in your life. Synchronicity falls at your doorstep. Unfortunately for most of us, it's not until we've gone through one or more crises that we even notice the door and begin to open it.

So why am I spending so much time in this chapter with what might seem like warnings? Because you are already wired to be aware of your intuition. It isn't difficult for you to develop it and begin using it ... but as sensitive people, we are also wired for very strong responses, worries about confrontation, and fears about doing the wrong thing. In other words, all the hiccups I mentioned above are going to come up. I want to save you as much frustration as possible, so that you can be the bright, shining, intuitive light that you are. I've tried to make Lethoso and the bunny debacle story as memorable as possible. Keep this chapter in mind and refer back to it often.

Getting Started with Intuition

As you hopefully deduced from my story, intuition is all about stepping just outside the way we normally think and worry. Our intuition is always there within us, but it is a separate system from our typical thoughts and emotional daydreaming. Therefore, to get started with intuition, I find it most helpful to do something that is completely different from thinking and feeling in the way we normally do. A great example of that is a practice called muscle testing or kinesiology.

The terms *kinesiology* and *muscle testing* mean various things to different types of health practitioners, but for our purpose of getting acquainted with our inner wisdom I define muscle testing as feeling how our intuition communicates electrochemically through our physical body. We return to this concept from our discussion way back in chapter 2, when we identified how we are vibrating, electrochemical beings. Now we'll experience that in a fun way that demonstrates the physical feedback of our intuition and inner wisdom.

. . . .

Muscle Testing "Yes–No" Intuition Exercise

Stand or sit with good posture and your feet flat on the floor. With your less-dominant hand touch the tip of your thumb to your pinky finger, making a circle. I'll refer to this thumb to littlest finger placement as "circle" for the rest of this exercise. By touching your fingers like this, you are creating an electrical circuit for your body to communicate with you.

With your dominant hand (the hand you write and do most things with) touch your thumb to your first (index) finger. I think of this as being like the head of a pair of pliers, which you can open and close. I will refer to this thumb to index finger placement as "pliers" for the rest of this exercise. With the pliers closed, insert those fingers into the circle you've made with your other hand. Notice that if you open the pliers wide, it breaks open the circle.

You will be able to feel your inner wisdom's answers to yes–no questions with this method by how much resistance the circle gives to the pliers. When your body is in agreement with you, or the answer is yes, a strong circuit is created. The pliers will have a very tough time breaking open the circle. If your body doesn't agree, or the answer is no, then the circuit is weakened. The circle will come apart very easily when you open the pliers.

Try this now with your name vs. a name that is not yours. Take a breath in to make sure you are centered and balanced. Insert the closed pliers into the circle. Say, "My name is (*insert your name here*)." Then open the pliers and feel the resistance. Now reset the pliers and circle and say, "My name is Floyd (*or any name that is not yours*)" and notice the difference when you open the pliers this time. Practice this a couple more times with simple yes–no statements, such as, I live in Minnesota vs. I live in (*insert your home state here*); I have brown eyes vs. I have blue eyes.

As you practice this, every once in a while you may not get a clear answer. Here are times that may happen:

- You are coming down with a cold or are otherwise ill.
- You phrased the question in an unclear way. There really isn't a preferable option between the two choices you've presented.
- You are distracted when asking the question. Even simple things can throw off your ability to easily communicate with your body, such as needing to use the bathroom or being too hungry. If you are fairly centered and undistracted, though, as you learn this technique, your body will communicate with you as clearly as it can.

I've found that this muscle testing technique is a great way for people to begin to get in touch with their intuition and the sometimes subtle way it communicates. It's a fun way to build trust with yourself. That's the biggest stumbling block I've noticed that people have to overcome—trust.

People are full of questions about intuition like, "How do I know I'm hearing my intuition vs. my own thoughts? How do I know when I can trust it?" This physical process circumvents those worries, so it is a good way to get started and build trust in yourself and your own inner wisdom, which will apply to intuition development and connecting with your empathic sensitivity.

Building Trust with Muscle Testing

This muscle testing technique can give you much more information than a simple yes or no. Here are some other ways to use muscle testing to give your inner wisdom a chance to communicate with you:

- The next time you are at a restaurant, ask yourself which item you should order, then do the circle/pliers for each item down the menu until you hit a really strong yes resistance. With this technique, people often find that they try new menu items they wouldn't normally have ordered, and they are delicious.
- When trying to decide between two different brands of oatmeal (or anything else) at the grocery store ask, "Which will be best for me?" then muscle test. Again, people sometimes find they try a new brand, and like it even better than what they had been buying.
- Let's say you are feeling exhausted. Before making a decision about what to do, ask yourself, "Will I feel better if I take a nap or take a walk?" It shouldn't be surprising that your body knows exactly what you should do to feel better.

Remember that how you phrase your question is important. If you are most concerned about which oatmeal will be the yummiest, then ask that. If you are more concerned about how it will make you feel, then ask, "Which oatmeal will give me the most energy from breakfast?" And if that is your question, you'll want to add a third choice: "What food will help me feel most energized after breakfast? This oatmeal? That oatmeal? Or some other food?" If you aren't getting a clear answer, then you may need to add the "something else" choice.

Have fun using this muscle testing technique to ask all sorts of questions about anything and any area of your life where you could use some helpful inner guidance. It's the simple questions that often will give your mind "proof" that you can communicate with your inner wisdom and intuition.

Making Friends with Your Empathic Sensitivity

Noticing and understanding your empathic ability is similar to following your intuition, but there are some distinct differences. The first
commonality is the importance of mindfulness, simply being present in
the current moment right now so you can be aware of the subtle flashes
of intuitive and empathic feelings. So if you skipped or only scanned
chapter 7, go back to it now and actually do the mindfulness exercises.
It is an imperative part of intuitive and psychic development.

The primary difference that leaves many sensitive people feeling
adversarial about their empathic ability is the pure emotional nature
of it. Intuition is a "knowing," so it is devoid of emotion. It just is.
Empathic ability, on the other hand, is pure, sometimes raw, emotional energy, and it can initially leave us overwhelmed, as in my story
in the introduction.

It is important to make friends with your empathic sensitivity. If
you are sensitive, you are empathic as well. It's sad to feel adversarial
toward something that is such a significant part of who you are. Empathic ability is meant to be useful. It really is, and it definitely can be.
In the past fifteen years, I have come a long, long, long way from the
empathic young psychologist in my story. At that time, I was overwhelmed by my empathic ability, had no idea how to modulate it, and
you had better believe I was very distraught about it. Empathic ability
and I were definitely not friends at that point in time.

Now, I fully recognize that it is simply part of the body, mind,
spirit totality of my sensitivity. Through flower essence therapy and
ardent practice developing my intuition and metaphysical senses, my
empathic ability is less intense because it is more refined.

Do I still "feel stuff" from clients? The answer is yes, but in a different way. For me, if the empathic energy I feel is not at all similar to
anything I am feeling, then it comes across as information that feels
very separate from who I am—it's more like intuition.

On the other hand, if the client's current crisis is very similar to
what I am also going through around that time, then I do indeed feel
it more directly. It sometimes is expressed in my dreams, sometimes

in emotional feelings or urges. Is that a problem? No, because it always, and I do mean always, leads me to the obvious path for healing and spiritual development that will benefit both my client *and* myself. My empathic ability shows me how my own emotions are similar and then shines a light on the way to heal that emotional discord in myself and in my client.

Empathic ability is, after all, not an invasion. It is a reminder that we are all connected. We are all stumbling through trying to do our best in this human condition, and as such, we all go through similar emotional experiences. We can all help each other, and we can all learn from each other.

And that is the crux of it. Empathic ability probably is going to be quite uncomfortable for you if you are not willing to honestly look at your own emotional baggage and begin to walk the path of self-evolution.

I imagine some of you are annoyed with me right now because your empathic ability is overwhelming, and you say, "I *am* trying, Dr. Kyra, and it still hurts too much!" Just keep on it. Try flower essences and other methods to help bring your empathic sensitivity into alignment.

In general, we aren't comfortable in our society with emotion, anyway, so to add empathic emotion on top of it can sometimes feel like too much. Be sure that you have read chapters 2 and 3 about empathic sensitivity to feel grounded about what exactly it is. If you are in the midst of being confused or sometimes annoyed with empathic emotion you are sensing, please reread chapter 5 about flower essence therapy and Appendix A: Another Perspective on Being Empathic by my colleague Molly Sheehan.

. . . .

Combining Muscle Testing and the Solar Plexus Meditation

For this activity, choose a feeling that is bothering you right now. It can be anything: sadness, apathy, frustration, etc. We are going to combine the muscle testing technique from the intuition section with the empathic solar plexus meditation from the end of chapter 2 to gain clarity about the sources of the bothersome feeling and what you can do about it.

Sit comfortably with good posture and your feet flat on the floor. Take in a slow, deep breath and exhale. Now bring up this feeling you want to know more about. Really feel it and notice where you feel it most in your body. We are going to ask the following questions: Is this feeling my own emotion? Is this feeling something I am picking up empathically from someone? Or is it some of both?

Now make the circle with your less-dominant pinky and thumb and the pliers with your dominant thumb and index finger. Bring up the feeling, insert the pliers into the circle, and ask, Is this feeling my own emotion? *Note if the answer is yes, no, or if there is medium resistance, the answer may be unclear or some of both. No matter the answer, repeat the process with the next two questions:* Is this feeling something I am picking up empathically from someone? Or is it some of both?

If you received the answer that there is an empathic component to the feeling either with a yes or some of both, we'll now do the solar plexus meditation to ask for more information about the feeling.

Now relax your hands and sit comfortably. Close your eyes and turn your attention to the part of your body that is just below your chest but above your abdomen. Remember that this area is called the solar plexus. This area is that network of nerves that connects to every internal organ in your body. It is your emotional, empathic nerve center.

Go within your body and really feel connected to your solar plexus… Now bring up the feeling you just asked about. Feel it centered in your solar plexus… And now ask What do I need to know about this empathic emotion? *Notice the very first thing that occurs to you, no matter how subtle it is, whether or not it makes any sense at the moment. Just notice the response, be it visual, a feeling, words, or just an impression…* What do I need to know about this empathic emotion? … *If you need further clari-*

fication about it, you can ask Where am I picking up this empathic emotion from? *Again, accept whatever impression occurs to you.*

You can still do this process even if your answer was that the feeling is your own emotion. It will be like doing your own inner wisdom counseling session. Follow the meditation connecting to your solar plexus and bring up the feeling, then ask the following questions: What do I need to know about this feeling? What would help shift and heal this feeling? *Remember in empathic meditation like this that it is best to keep your questions as open as possible. That's why we ask,* What do I need to know? *Then you are not limiting the answers that your inner wisdom can give back to you.*

Although you think you'll remember, it's a good idea to immediately draw or write down the answers you received to your questions. In fact, I recommend you keep a journal for these experiences as you learn about your empathic ability and intuition. You'll want to refer back to it later. Oftentimes when we fall back into our usual thought patterns, we forget the intuitive information we received and the helpful guidance it may have given us.

If you don't receive clear answers when you connect to your solar plexus, don't fret. This may be the first time you have ever tried anything like this, and it simply may take a little practice. As you continue learning about your empathic ability, and continue with intuition development, you *will* get there. It will change. If you decide to make friends with your empathic ability, to respect it, and to use the information it is giving you for your benefit (just like intuition), then I guarantee 100 percent, it will evolve and change as you do. It will become more refined and beneficial, and you will become clearer and lighter as you allow the energetic part of your sensitivity to guide you.

Sooner or later, you will find that all your sensitivities in body, mind, and spirit allow you to fully experience the world in very positive ways. The more you clear and heal, the more your sensitivities pick up on all the good stuff: beauty, positivity, "good luck," and amazing experiences are waiting for every sensitive person.

CHAPTER 9

Enjoying the Best Life
Has to Offer

Most of us have learned to cope with our sensitivity by making our world smaller—limiting sensory input, avoiding potential conflicts, and generally reducing the opportunities available to us. But what if we've had it backward the whole time? What if being sensitive is an indication that we are meant to relish every single thing the world offers in a big way? What if it means that we have an expansive capability to experience wonderful things with our keen senses and love every moment of life? It wouldn't be the first time common "wisdom" had everything backward.

I mean, think about it. Why would we have these abilities to feel what others cannot, to appreciate what others don't, and to savor even the subtlest sensory joys far more than the average person? We're obviously built to enjoy life and to partake of every sensory pleasure in a big way. We're the ones who resonate with the earth and all her flora and fauna. We're designed to really *live* this life as a vibrant, colorful, rich sensory experience on every level of our being.

Also why would we have such empathy and compassion? We're the ones who care exponentially. We're the humans who will fix the messes humanity has made by being able to sense and see the solutions that are only found outside the box of conventional thought. Is it no wonder then that our children are being born with more inherent sensitivities? They will need them in order to bring humanity and the earth back around to a place of harmony and respect.

On this theme, let's discuss a phrase that is very commonly used, yet its meaning is often left obscure. Most people are familiar with the Bible verse, "Blessed are the meek, for they shall inherit the earth."[20] It's such a well-known verse, yet who can explain what it really means? I'm sure there are many different interpretations to be found, but it's a simple statement that doesn't require over-analyzing.

Blessed = divinely revered

Meek = gentle, sensitive

Inherit = to come into possession of or receive, especially as a right or a divine portion

The earth = our home, our cultures, and our societies, and all the splendor and greatest sensory stuff about living in this world, as in the Garden of Eden

Thank heavens for the *sensitive people* for they shall *receive in divine portion* the *society we live in and all the best things about living on earth.*

In other words, divine wisdom has always acknowledged our importance in earth's destiny.

The less sensitive have had the lion's share of control over society and earth's resources for quite a while now, so the time has come for us to spread our sensitive influence and take back our portion, as is our divine right. We need to snap out of our complacency and know it is not our place to accept less.

---

20. The Official King James Bible Online, *King James Bible "Authorized Version" Cambridge Edition*, "Matthew 5:5," accessed August 1, 2015, http://www.kingjames bibleonline.org/Matthew-5-5.

I'm not the only one feeling this pull. I love to hear and read of obviously sensitive people taking a stand and reclaiming their energetic space.

I recently read a fabulous blog article that illustrates this point as directly as I have ever seen.[21] It's also hilarious. (Warning: There is a bit of frank language contained in her post. Don't say I didn't warn you.) The setup for this story is as follows: Cassie is a hard-working, sensitive young woman who has two jobs. She rides the New York City subway daily. One day she finally became fed up with what she calls "manspreaders," guys who sit with their legs spread wide, taking up two or three seats, oblivious to everyone else, even on a very crowded train.

Cassie describes how these guys think they are the center of the universe "never once considering the lady with the stroller, the World War II vet stooped over a cane, or the child riding home from school alone."

She continues, "We all go about our ride politely avoiding calling them out on their selfishness, holding grocery bags and diaper bags and the weight of all our frustration."

And then it happened, in a moment of clarity, Cassie said it dawned on her that being frustrated doesn't help anyone, but "sitting on a dude" sure would be satisfying. And for the very first time she announced, "Excuse me," and SAT ON A GUY'S THIGH!

The thigh that was carelessly placed between Cassie and her train seat became a non-obstacle. She sat on him, and do you know what happened? Do you think he got angry or confronted her? Nope, exactly the opposite. Cassie comically describes how she never saw anyone react so quickly to get out of the way. She took the space that rightfully was due to her, and it felt good.

---

21. Cassie J. Sneider, XO Jane Blog, "I Have Been Sitting on Manspreaders For the Last Month and I Have Never Felt More Free: How I Snapped and Started Taking Up as Much Space as I Deserve," accessed June 6, 2015, http://www.xojane.com /issues/sitting-on-manspreaders.

She has continued her manspreader sitting practice, claiming her space. In true sensitive, caring person style, Cassie ends her story with, "Let's sit down *together*."

Notice that she didn't take away anything from anyone. Rather, Cassie is teaching us to advocate for the space we deserve, while she is also showing the less sensitive that they will be just fine moving over. There is room enough for everyone in this world. We can share.

If you've made it this far, then you've no doubt noticed how much I love metaphors. This manspreading story is the greatest metaphor I've ever encountered to illustrate the energetic shift that is happening between the sensitive community and the less-sensitive populace. Please believe that the less-sensitive people and parts of the world are no longer in our way.

Shortly after I read the manspreading blog article, I had a chance to practice something similar. I was sitting in my car at a gas pump at a gas station. I remembered that I had a coupon in my e-mail, so I was fiddling with my phone for several minutes to try to find it. I looked up and noticed in my rear view mirror that a guy in a car had pulled up behind me and was obviously waiting for me to move so he could pull his car up to the pump.

Because I'm sensitive, I can sense the energetic pressure of someone behind me, and I often experience this while driving, so I'm not surprised I felt it in this instance. In the past, this is how I would have reacted, "Oh, this guy's waiting for me. I better hurry up and move. He looks annoyed so I don't want to make the situation worse." I used to be more than willing to inconvenience myself for someone else's comfort.

But, I looked around and counted. There were twenty gas pumps at this station. Twenty! And some of them were open. So this guy had nineteen other options, at least three of them clearly better choices than sitting behind me, because they were entirely available. I decided to own my space and time. I left my car exactly where it was at the pump, got out of my car, and started walking to the convenience store to use my coupon where I would pay ahead for my gas as I had originally planned.

In the past, I definitely would have changed my plans and used my credit card to fill my car up as quickly as possible and get out of his way.

Was he mad that I kept him waiting? Oh, yes. As I walked to the convenience shop, he zoomed off in his car and yelled, "As*hole!" at me. And my reaction? I was at peace in total clarity that the situation was his doing. For whatever reason that didn't matter to me, he was being stubborn and oblivious. He could have easily moved his car to an open pump.

Now, of course, use your intuition about the safety of any similar situation you may find yourself in. I wasn't being a jerk. If it had been a small gas station with no open pumps, I would have reacted differently based on that situation. But what I am saying is that every small claim we make grows and grows, making it easier to ultimately "inherit the earth," as is our birthright.

The time is perfect, right now, for sensitive people to edge in. We should never apologize for being here and expecting to be treated fairly, with compassion for all involved.

Although you may question it sometimes, the world at large is changing and becoming more sensitively aware. In North American society, there are very strong pushes for compassion and more awareness of things like better treatment toward animals, social justice and equality, organic and safer foods, and truth in labeling.

We have affected commerce. Fragrance-free products are available on store shelves. Chemical-free foods are marketed to us on a regular basis now. And if you say, "Well, that's just business. Companies only make what sells," then I would answer, "Yes. We are claiming our piece of the capitalistic pie, which is growing and growing."

But what about all the other terrible, chemical-filled products and food-coloring filled convenience foods? They are still there. Please remember the metaphor of Cassie's subway train story. We don't need *every* seat on the train. Cassie didn't run through the subway car sitting on everybody. She only took what was rightfully her space to have. As she said, we can all "sit together."

As we, the sensitive, perceptive, and aware segment of the population, claim our space, exercise our rights, make our preferences known, and *expect* to be treated respectfully, then the rest of society will simply have to adapt. And they will.

· · · · · · · · · · ·

We have covered a lot of ground in these chapters. The reason I wrote this book was so people would know that there is so much more to their sensitivity than the physical and emotional discomforts that common thought dictate. We are energetic beings as well. Misunderstood and ignored empathic ability creates a huge gap in understanding who we truly are as sensitive, perceptive people. In fact, this disregard for all things metaphysical often leads to unnecessary depression and emotional suffering.

I hope this book will help many sensitive people stop blaming themselves and retreating from life to minimize their discomforts. Rather, it is time for us to step forward and expand our definition of who we are as highly perceptive, sensitive individuals. We have many abilities and gifts to embrace, especially when we consider all that we are in body, mind, and spirit.

My hope is that the new perspectives and tools in this book will change the life of every sensitive person who is struggling with overwrought emotions and low self-worth. No one should suffer for being empathic. Our capacity for empathy is the stuff of life. It is a demonstration of all humans' connection to one another. It is our energetic heart telling us what we need to know to heal ourselves. And as we do that, we heal others and we heal the earth without even having to try. Many people refer to sensitive souls as "lighthouses," meaning that we shine a beacon of light that helps others find their way. You don't have to be a doctor or a counselor or a healer of any profession to do that. All you have to do is be who you are. Sensitive people are important in this world. *You* are important in this world.

Keen perception, creativity, intuitive senses, and empathy are strengths that most everyone in this world secretly covets whether they admit to it or not. When we are balanced, then we have all of these strengths at our disposal. So what I've aimed to do is provide that balance. I've selected each new way of thinking, every exercise, every holistic tool in this book precisely for you so you can create that balance in your life. The strengths of your sensitivity are already within you, and the process is about uncovering them to allow them to shine.

Last but not least, I want every sensitive person to claim his or her right to be here, to fully experience everything rewarding about this life, and to be happy. Can you imagine a world in which every sensitive person lives that way? I can, and it shifts the energy of the entire earth in unpredictably positive ways.

Another Perspective on Being Empathic

by Molly Sheehan of Green Hope Farm

Note from Dr. Kyra: I've come to know Molly Sheehan as the creator of lovely, high-vibration flower essences. Molly always communicates in a clear, down-to-earth manner and is up front about what she herself has experienced and continues to learn. She is a sensitive soul who has dedicated her life to cocreating healing energies with nature. She understands, in great depth, the support we all need in our path of self-evolution. Molly helped me years ago after an illness left my sensitivities raw and overwhelmed. In other words, Molly knows her stuff. I hope you will also appreciate her perspective on being empathic.

· · · · · · · · · · ·

There are many gifts and challenges to being an empath. Here's some of what I have learned about being an empath, about validating my empathic skills, and how to take better care of myself as an empathic person.

What Is an Empath?

Being empathic is one way to describe a general ability to sense what people are feeling without conventional methods of information gathering. In other words, empaths often know what another person is feeling, even when the other person doesn't tell or show them this.

Empaths often have very accurate information without any conventional explanation for how they know what they know. Sometimes this extends to knowing what is going on physiologically for people, as well as knowing how they are feeling emotionally.

Empaths take an ability that lies latent in all of us—the ability to read each other's energy field—and develop this into a skill set. Some people are born more empathic than others, but often times this skill set is improved through conscious as well as unconscious use.

There are many reasons someone might develop this skill set. First, let's look at the situation for empathic children and why they might hone their empathic skills.

Growing Up Empathic

In general, growing up as an empath can be confusing. It is particularly confusing when an empathic child knows what people are feeling, but these emotions remain unacknowledged by the people feeling them.

Another confusing aspect of being an empathic child is that adults often do not acknowledge it is possible that a person can empathically sense what other people are feeling. This can make an empathic child feel lonely and anxious that he or she is imagining things.

Even when no one acknowledges these skills, many empathic kids develop their empathic skills anyway. One motivation for developing these empathic skills is a self-protective one. Take a common situation in which what is said in a family is out of alignment with what actually happens in the family. An example of this might be parents talking about what a harmonious and happy family they are, when the adults are actually unhappy and take this out on their children through abusive behaviors. Empathic children find that in order to be prepared for what the adults in their life are actually going to do, versus what they say they are going to do, it helps them to hone their empathic skills and listen to the emotional subtext.

Empathic children zero in on this split between what people say and how they feel because it can help them be slightly more prepared for unpleasant events. However, this split between how adults talk about the world and how empathic children experience it can be very difficult for the child.

No matter who we are, it is important to have some other person validate our experiences. However, for an empathic child, the adults in his or her life may be unable to understand or validate their child's abilities. This leaves the child with the choice to either cut off from this empathic part or cut off and hide this part of him- or herself from the people who deny those empathic gifts.

People may have benign motivations for questioning an empathic child's experiences. They may not be aware that anyone can empathically know what another is feeling, and therefore they believe they are helping an empath by talking her out of her insights. Other times however, parents of an empath may not be ready to look honestly at the situation that their child is seeing more clearly. Peers of an empath may not want to admit what a cutthroat situation they find themselves in socially. There are many reasons parents, peers, or other people may be unable or unwilling to validate a child's empathic experiences.

I love knowing there are empathic children who have parents accepting their empathic experiences and acknowledging them as legitimate and real. What a wonderful way to develop one's empathic skill set—because a parent or a mentor is acknowledging it and holding it to be authentic and valuable.

I suspect most adult empaths have not had this kind of childhood and therefore have a complicated set of issues to resolve in adulthood.

Being an Adult Empath After a Childhood without Validation

Empaths who were dismissed or even blamed during their childhoods often have a difficult time trusting their own instincts as adults. While they may have developed excellent empathic skills, they won't necessarily back up their sixth sense. Why? Because they have had no model for this process.

Empaths have often been at the receiving end of personalities who would rather have them not mention what they know. This means the self-edit button and the self-judgment button are often well developed and overused by empaths. It is a worthwhile but challenging process to begin to validate what our empathic self knows.

After all, empaths have accumulated a lot of shaming experiences in which other people have told them they are imagining other people's negativity. They often come to the conclusion that any negativity they sense must be their own.

It is a big understatement to say that many empaths believe that everything they are feeling is their own stuff. They usually have had no one offer them the understanding that a lot of the feelings they experience are from moving through other people's energetic or electrical fields and *do not* belong to them. In fact, as I mentioned before, they probably have had a lot of experiences in which people told them the feelings *did* belong to them.

This confusion about who owns what can be a consequence of growing up in a household where empathic skills are not recognized. If, as a child, there is a lot of emotional business not being acknowledged in a household, the empathic child *still* feels these unacknowledged feelings. A few instances in which an empathic child mentions whatever is going on and gets told that she is imagining things can leave this child with a lifelong tendency to take everything on. Once this pattern gets set, it's not a leap before the person believes if all the emotions are her emotions, then all the clean up is hers also.

I am sure that there are lots of other complicated factors here, but what it all boils down to is that most empaths *have a pattern of feeling responsible for everything they feel.* This can set up a lifelong pattern of confusion about whose business *any* problem is.

In the best of all possible worlds, a child learns that her empathic gifts are real, and also this important point: Sometimes it is appropriate to do something with her insight, but oftentimes there is nothing that she needs to do with what she knows but acknowledge it and *let it go.*

How to Heal the Confusion

It is a terrible burden to feel responsible for cleaning up so many feelings, but it is also a logical conclusion to draw when the adults in an empath's childhood deny all the emotions swirling about.

One fellow empath continually reminds me to be gentle with myself as I try to figure out which problems belong to whom. My own tendency has been to add insult to injury. When I realize I have taken on somebody else's emotional problem as my own, I don't just let go. I let go and then give myself a hard time about my confusion. It is important to realize that empaths live through intense situations without any guidance for how to handle these situations. As we learn management skills for our empathic insights, kindness to ourselves is necessary.

One difficulty that occurs when we think everything we feel is ours is that we tend to keep all the feelings in our own energy system versus watching them come and go without any sense of personal responsibility. This is very hard on our energy system and is something that negatively affects our health and well-being.

There are many reasons why carrying other people's emotions as our own does not help anyone. First, it prevents people from dealing with their own business. If an empath takes on another's energetic business, the empath prevents this person from getting on with the work of solving his own problems. But please no shame here! If you have a tendency to take on other people's emotions as your own, it is almost certainly because as a child you were encouraged to do so. As you get clear about why it is not helpful to do this, try to course correct without self-judgment!

Another profoundly important reason why it is not a good idea to take on other people's emotional business is that it wears on our electrical and physical systems to carry all this stuff that is not ours. It is fine to be helpful in any way we feel called to help, and then make sure we have cleared our own energetic fields and are no longer carrying anyone else's emotions or energetics in our fields.

I have had a lot of difficulties learning to be more meticulous about clearing my energy field. I had the usual confusion about who owned what emotions and often didn't realize what a spring cleaning I needed. It also took me years to realize I needed to ask my inner wisdom if it was my job to take on other people's emotional business. This would seem to be a straightforward enough question with a straightforward enough *no* answer, but I often lapsed into the confused thinking of my childhood in which it worked for the adults around me to have me own their emotional garbage. It worked to cheer them up and in some way try and "fix" them. This is another part of the dynamic for an empath. We seem to attract people who are happy to have us carry their emotional stuff for them. It is a challenge to remember that our intellects may not make the wisest decision about who should carry the emotional baggage in any situation. Our divine selves do a better job of knowing that we all need to carry our own stuff and no one else's.

As a young adult, I had a dramatic learning lesson in a situation in which no one was asking me to carry anything for them. I thought because I could read the energy of a gathering of people, it was my job to "fix" their energetics. There were many problems with my process, including the idea that there was anything to fix in the first place.

Early in my career, I was giving a talk to a couple hundred people at the annual American Dowsing Convention in Vermont. This was before I had much practice seeing my own patterns of over-responsibility at work or had any tools to shift my patterns. But let me tell you, did this experience ever motivate me to learn some new tricks!

Dowsers are incredible networkers and information gatherers, but they don't always take the time to ground what they are learning into their bodies. At their annual convention, many dowsers walk around with so much mental energy and new information collected above their heads that it's amazing they can stand up. As I began my talk to the convention, I sensed the ungrounded nature of the crowd and decided, without being asked and without checking with my own guidance, to "help" them out by grounding all the mental energy for them through myself.

I don't exactly know what I did or exactly why I did it, but I sure experienced consequences for my decision. I walked into my talk in good health and after my "helpful" gesture, I staggered out of the meeting hall with full blown pneumonia. *Whoa!* Talk about a wake-up call!

A year later, when I returned to speak to this group again, I went with trepidation. I had thought a lot about the event during the intervening year, but I wasn't completely convinced I had figured out what had happened or how I could correct it. I didn't want to live frightened of such situations, so I knew I had to go back and try again. I had to see if I had learned anything during my year of searching for answers.

First of all, I realized there was nothing wrong with the crowd. They were just being their curious selves. I also realized that their ungroundedness was their business. But my empathic nature made it difficult for me not to tune in to this ungroundedness and click into my pattern of "fixing" this, because I did not like the feeling of such ungroundedness myself.

I decided to begin my talk with a guided meditation in which I gave everybody a chance to ground themselves. This gave them a free will opportunity to ground or not. I tried not to move any energies through my own body. I also offered a sunflower flower essence to anyone who wanted to take it to help with this grounding process. I decided to try not to feel into the energy of the crowd in any way, shape, or form, but just give my talk and then let go.

It was a moment of satisfaction, relief, and gratefulness as I walked out of the talk in good health. I cannot tell you that I never goofed up again during the years I was out talking to large crowds, because I did, but this was a moment of proving to myself that I had learned something!

Additional things I would do now in the same circumstance include using grounding or clearing flower essences or taking a brief moment for myself afterward to do a meditation to clear my energy field (see Appendix C: Meditations for Sensitive People for an example of a clearing meditation).

One Final Thought

Sometimes it is not so simple to keep our energy field clear, even when we may think we are being detached or letting go. In my own life, I sometimes need to examine my patterns in conversation in order to see my confused thinking and get the *ah-ha* moment that helps me to let go of someone else's stuff.

One thing I have to watch for in myself is that I often pick up the energies of people who remind me of some of the adults from my childhood. Their archetypal behavior can trigger my old responses of over-responsibility. Sometimes it is not enough to remind myself of the logic of a situation. Yes, I know it is better for someone to take care of his or her own emotional business, but my own patterns can get activated subconsciously. This is why I try to check my system regularly to see where I am still holding on. Sometimes it takes a while to let stuff in my field go, but staying aware, using flower essences, meditating, and checking in with my inner guidance helps. As I see the patterns in my daily life more clearly, I become more aware of any lingering energetics that are not mine to clear from my field. This is an ongoing process.

For all the difficulties with being empathic, there are also the amazing gifts of being able to feel what it is like to walk in another's shoes. This can open such floodgates of love and oneness. I am most grateful for these experiences. Empathic skills are infinitely precious. They are skills we need to honor, acknowledge, and support!

APPENDIX B

Resources for Flower Essences

This list is just a small sample of some of the flower essence resources across the world, with information about a few of their most relevant essences for sensitivity. Yarrow does not grow in all climates. If you do not see yarrow or a sensitivity mixture listed under any of the following flower essence manufacturers, contact them and ask what they offer that is similar.

United States

FES (Flower Essence Services)
>   fesflowers.com
>   800-548-0075
>   Nevada City, California

FES essences are sold in many co-ops and health stores around the country. Check the FES website to see if they are available in your area.

Angelica—Awareness of spiritual guidance at times of stress or during overwhelming feelings of aloneness; positive spiritual sensitivity that allows one to feel protected and "seen."

Calendula—True perception and sensitivity in listening to another; allowing warm, nurturing communication with others; ability to hold one's thinking and speech back in order to "hear" another.

Chamomile—Subject to emotional tension and easily fluctuating moods; cries easily or feels minor aches and pains out of proportion to actual impact.

Chaparral—Absorption of disturbing or violent images, either from direct experience or mass media; toxic memories that overwhelm the consciousness due to prior trauma.

Desert Lily—Pronounced sensitivity leading to depletion stemming from the chaos of urban technological culture; deep desire in the soul for harmony and beauty; usually used in tandem with YES (Yarrow Environmental Solution).

Golden Yarrow—To address active involvement in life despite acute sensitivity; professional activities such as an artist or teacher that require performance for others despite innate sensitivity.

Lavender—Intense spiritual activity and resultant sensitivity accompanied by nervous characteristics, such as excess movement, fidgeting, light sleep, or insomnia.

Love-Lies-Bleeding—Intense personal suffering, either psychic or physical that overwhelms the soul; ability to accept and transform pain through compassionate awareness for oneself or others.

Mountain Pennyroyal—For energetic hygiene; works as a purgative to cleanse and expel negativity or other intrusions; clarifies the mental and etheric bodies, leading to increased vitality.

Mugwort—To develop greater sensitivity for one's dream life and its connection to active, awake daytime consciousness; general sleep aid.

Nicotiana—Masking sensitivity with a strong, tough exterior and emotional numbness as a way of coping with one's feelings; provides assistance to quit smoking.

Pink Monkeyflower—Extreme sensitivity resulting from abuse, body-shaming, or related cultural or familial experiences; inability to show or express one's real feelings due to profound feelings of unworthiness or feeling unloved or unwanted.

Pink Yarrow—Oversensitivity to the emotions of others; internalizing others' problems as one's own.

Purple Monkeyflower—Sensitivity characterized by fear of spiritual phenomena in particular; hypersensitivity and fear leading to unbalanced psychic experiences.

Saint John's Wort—Over-expanded, ungrounded psyche; vulnerability to environmental stress and allergies; especially indicated for disturbed sleep or dreams, nighttime sweating or bed-wetting; useful for seasonal affective disorder.

Star Tulip—Openness to spiritual realms; inner receptivity; helps with meditation.

Yarrow—Sensitivity to others and the environment; easily depleted; feeling overly absorbent of negative influences; increases inner radiance and strength.

Yarrow Environmental Solution (YES formula)*—This mixture, containing yarrow, echinacea, and arnica flower essences, is designed to enhance our energetic integrity to balance environmental toxins such as electromagnetic radiation, pollution, and residual effects from past exposure.

*Note from Dr. Kyra: Many of my readers have purchased Yarrow Environmental Solution (YES), thinking it was just a combination of yarrows and would work the same way as the individual yarrow essences. It does not. YES is for environmental and related physical sensitivities, particularly to radiation and EMF. Stick to the individual yarrow, pink yarrow, or golden yarrow essences for overall recalibration of your sensitivity.

Green Hope Farm

www.greenhopeessences.com
603-469-3662
Meriden, New Hampshire

Green Hope essences are preserved with vinegar and red shiso, rather than alcohol.

Golden Armor—Golden Armor is a mixture of yarrow and several golden flowers. It provides information to our electrical systems about how to buffer and protect us from computer screens, radiation, and atmospheric changes, human negativity, dissonant sounds, viruses, bacteria, man-made dissonance in the airwaves, and any other kind of vibrational bombardment we experience.

Grounding—Made from many tree flower essences and other deeply rooted flowering plants, Grounding is all about helping us to be here now, fully grounded and engaged in our lives.

Lamb's Ear—Lamb's ear essence communicates a way of balance in which a sensitive soul can know the finest nuance of a situation but also stay strong. No wilting away here.

Pink Yarrow from the Cliffs of Moher—Like the dramatic Cliffs of Moher in Ireland where this essence was made, this pink yarrow essence has a vibration of confident splendor, complete ease, and unapologetic self-expression. The essence encourages us to shine in all our glory even when we are in a place of extreme exposure or vulnerability.

Saint John's Wort—Offers tremendous wisdom about protection. It does not take up combat with external forces so much as help us remember the shining golden armor of light that we already wear. It teaches us that strong, protective golden light permeates our entire being and is our essential nature and birthright. Once discovered and claimed, this light easily protects us from environmental negativity, negative thought forms, or any firestorms around us.

White Yarrow—White yarrow protects us from anything that might disrupt the smooth electrical functioning of our energy systems.

Wing Span of the Senses—From Green Hope's Healer's Toolbox essences, the Wing Span of the Senses allows us to be open as we partake in healing and humanitarian work but also stay grounded in our own energy field. It helps us work deeply with another but not become tangled in their energetic field and/or current situation.

Babies of Light—The wise and sensitive souls coming to earth right now need help to adjust to the dissonant man-made vibrations they face. This essence offers necessary electrical protection and also helps them build their own protective electrical buffer.

Violet Transmuting Flame—Helps us permanently erase negativity from our energy systems without the balancing of karmic events. It can also be used to cleanse any part of earth and all her inhabitants.

Thistle from Omey Island—The protective energies of thistle get an Irish twist, specifically offering support to close down energy leaks caused by our reactions to people or circumstances passing out of our lives for any reason.

Alaskan Essences

alaskanessences.com
800-545-9309
Victor, Montana

All of the following can be found at the Alaskan Essences website under "Research Essences."

Alaska Violet—Supports those who feel overcautious, timid, reticent, and unable to actualize their life purpose in a practical way on the physical plane. For finding the right energetic relationship with others, especially in crowded situations.

Alpine Arnica—Helps us let go of our accumulation of past hurts without going through every detail of what happened and why; promotes ease, deep calm, and balance.

Bleeding Heart—For those who feel rejected by the self, heart closed to others, or lack of compassion for ourselves; promotes loving kindness to self and others.

Lavender Yarrow—Gives strength and protection to the higher chakras; heals the depletion that results from a chaotic influx of energy through the crown chakra.

Pasque Flower—For sensitive people who are uncomfortable with physical contact or lose their sense of self in crowded or intimate situations. Pasque helps create and maintain security through functional energy boundaries; helps us feel respected, appreciated, and protected.

Stinging Nettle—Helps those who are highly sensitive stay connected to earth and to their feelings; heals alienation in those who have been hurt deeply and have a tendency to repel those they want to be close to; promotes grounding and reconnection after being overwhelmed by too much input.

Featherhawk Essences

featherhawk.com

877-226-7858

New Albany, Indiana

Nanci Wesling, owner of Featherhawk, is very knowledgeable about sensitivity and offers workshops in her area. She has created a unique mixture called Yarrow Blend, which contains four types of yarrow plus white clover. She offers a choice of red shiso or alcohol as the preservative.

Click "Essences for Highly Sensitive People" at featherhawk.com to be taken to a list of fifteen essences including corn, various yarrows, sweetgrass, violet, and other remedies created by Nanci.

Yarrow Blend—Strengthens and maintains the integrity of your auric energy field, providing protection without armoring or creating an impenetrable wall. For maintaining a strong sense of self with appropriate emotional and energetic boundaries.

Freedom Flowers

freedom-flowers.com

208-935-5668

Kooskia, Idaho

Seneca Schurbon, the creator of Freedom Flower Essences, offers a free seven day e-course to teach you how to get started using flower essences.

Yarrow Shield Mixture—Beneficial for those who are sensitive to environments and other people's moods and energies. Especially recommended for those who are in healing or care-giving professions where the tendency is to take on what others are going through. Establishes safe boundaries and is protective against intentional attack or passive absorption. Contains five essences including yarrow, black locust, and rhubarb.

Australia

Living Essences of Australia
livingessences.com.au
+00 61 (0)8 9301 1234
Western Australia

Correa—Inspires feelings of positivity and self-esteem. Being able to learn from mistakes with acceptance and without blame or regret. Helpful for overcoming negative self-concepts.

Geraldton Wax—Inner strength and being true to yourself. To feel the beauty of being strong against the wind of adverse opinion and pressure. To strengthen oneself so as not to be pressured against one's will, or be routinely influenced by others' desires.

Inner Strength Blend—To counter depletion of vital force, being easily unbalanced by outside influences, needing resilience, swinging between high and low energy levels.

Parakeeyla—Self-esteem and assertiveness. For hardworking people who feel lonely and sad because they are unappreciated. This essence restores a sense of self-dignity and inner strength, not to withdraw, but to be an active part of society and able to assert one's rights as an individual.

Urchin Dryandra—Positive appreciation of one's internal gifts. Boosts self-worth and overcomes the role of victim in relationships; breaks up inferiority complexes.

Himalayan Flower Enhancers
himalaya.com.au
+61 2 4473 7131
New South Wales, Australia

Aura Cleaning—Cleans and refreshes the etheric body

Protection Mix—Protection from unwanted psychic, emotional energies.

Sober Up—Helps give balance and stability to people with a tendency toward drug and alcohol abuse and related problems.

Canada

Pacific Essences

pacificessences.com

+1 250-384-5560

Victoria, British Columbia

Pacific Essences offers Energy Medicine Cards which contains seventy-two cards of their flower and sea essences. They make interesting essences from sea life.

Balancer Mix—Use in times of stress and mental or emotional overload. It is particularly useful when we feel overwhelmed and unable to cope.

Canadian Forest Tree Essences

essences.ca

+1 819-319-6162

Gatineau, Quebec

Therapist & Healer Combination Mix—For those who are easily affected by crowds and other people's emotions; exhausted when surrounded by many people through the day; a tool for protection and clearing.

England

Bach Flower Remedies

bachcentre.com

+44 (0)1491 834678

Oxfordshire, UK

Offers information and education about the thirty-eight flower essences in the Bach remedy system, plus a practitioner locator with worldwide listings.

Aspen—For those who feel hypersensitive to things unseen or unknown; have vague anxiety and apprehension; need for psychic balance.

Red Chestnut—Over-concern and worry about the well-being of others; misplaced anxiety and worry which drains the soul forces.

Star of Bethlehem—Soothes acute sensitivity and trauma, especially post-trauma stress.

Walnut—Helps protect us against outside influences in general. Walnut people are fulfilling their purpose in life but sometimes doubt their path when they hear the opinions, theories, or beliefs of others. Also useful at all the transition points in life; helps us move forward.

Ireland

Living Frequencies
living-frequencies.com
00-353-402-35432
Cork, Ireland

Now Earth Yarrow—Use this essence when feeling vulnerable and in need of psychic protection. This feeling is often present when we are not fully and firmly anchored within ourselves.

Ursula Selwood also creates *flower essence digital art*, which offers the healing energy of flowers just by looking at it. You can find the images on the Living Frequencies website.

New Zealand

First Light Flower Essences of New Zealand
nzfloweressences.co.nz
+64 9 817-6737
Auckland, New Zealand

Fern Collection—Offers seven essences for overcoming and transcending abuse and trauma.

Healer's Collection—Lace Fern, Smooth Shield Fern, and Black Shield Fern all provide energetic recalibration for empathic people.

Orchid Collection—Features several essences specifically designed for sensitive children.

Scotland

Findhorn Flower Essences
findhornessences.com
+44 (0) 1309 690129
Morayshire, Scotland

Energy Shield Mix—Helps to purify, transform, and release negative energies and influences that are electromagnetic and emotional.

Psychic Protection Mix—Maintain your sense of safety and inner security; interact and socialize with others without absorbing negativity; set clear boundaries; stay positive and strong.

Sea Holly—Overcome your insecurities and inhibitions; step out boldly and express your thoughts, feelings, and ideas with confidence. Feel liberated and realize your full potential, standing in your power to be the radiant, enterprising, and brilliant being that you are.

South Africa

South African Flower Essences
safloweressences.co.za
+27-21-7946762
Cape Town, South Africa

Wild Sage—For those who are prone to absorbing negativity from others. Aligns the subtle bodies and draws in the will forces, enabling one to draw on spiritual strength and take back one's power. Often used in combination with yarrow.

Yarrow—Strengthens and stimulates the integrity of the aura. It is an important essence for stabilizing and buffering against negativity.

Guided Meditations for Sensitive People

Every meditation transcribed in this book is also available in audio file format at www.drkyra.com. I'm providing these written meditation scripts though so you can memorize them, record them yourself, or read them aloud to someone else. Each of these meditations begins with a different introduction to teach you various ways to quickly calm and focus.

. . . .

Grounding Tree Meditation

The purpose of this meditation is to bring you back down to earth when you are feeling overwhelmed with stress, like you have "frazzled nerves," or are having trouble focusing because you are feeling scattered. This is also a useful meditation to do anytime you feel the need to reconnect with nature, but it may not be accessible to you at the time due to winter or an urban environment.

Sit comfortably, feeling supported, with your arms relaxed, and your feet flat on the floor. Close your eyes and take in a deep, relaxing breath. We're going to focus for the first few moments on our breathing. On your next breath, when you breathe in count slowly to 2, pause, and then exhale slowly to the count of 2. Inhale 1 ... 2 pause ... exhale 1 ... 2. Good. Now we're going to gently breathe to the count of 3. Inhale 1 ... 2 ... 3 pause ... exhale 1 ... 2 ... 3. Notice how your body easily lets go as you breathe. Breathing to 3, even more slowly and relaxed this time. Breathe in 1 ... 2 ... 3 ... pause ... Breathing out 1 ... 2 ... and 3.

Now imagine a really huge, old tree. This might be a tree you have seen before or not. Any kind of tree that occurs to you is just fine ... So first just notice what type of tree it seems to be and what it looks like ... Also take in the surroundings. Where is this tree's home? What is the landscape like? What animals live in and around the tree? What other plants are in the area? Notice everything else about this beautiful place including the sky and the ground.

Listen for a moment to the sounds of this environment. Maybe you'll hear the breeze rustle the leaves in the tree. Are there sounds of birds or animals? Pause to take it all in.

What is the weather like in this place? Notice what you are wearing and what you feel against your skin including a gentle breeze or the warmth of the sun ...

Reach out and feel the bark of the tree. Place your hands on the trunk. You can actually feel the wise old earth energy of this tree pass from its trunk into your hands.

You glance down and notice a spot at the base of the tree where the roots are visible. It almost looks like the roots have formed a comfortable place to sit right up against the tree. So you take a seat and find that it is very comfortable ... Your back is against the trunk of the tree and the soft earth supports you.

Take in a deep breath and notice how fresh it smells as the tree shares fresh oxygen with you. You exhale and sense the tree's leaves absorbing your carbon dioxide. Notice this cycle for a few breaths. The tree's leaves send you oxygen, which you breathe in ... You exhale and the tree breathes in ... The tree exhales and you breathe in ... Exhaling and inhaling.

Then you become aware of the tree's roots underground. You realize that the tree must have a massive root system that extends far down into the earth. Your awareness follows the tree's roots out and down through the different layers of dirt and soil. Past the earthworms and moles that live in the earth... Where the roots pull in water and earth energy that travel back up the roots and up through the tree's trunk. The tree invites you to join the roots, so you feel that rooted, grounded energy travel up from the earth and up through your spine all the way up to the top of your head... Feeling that grounded earth energy, slow your breathing and clear your energy. You feel supported, grounded, and at one with the tree, the ground, and the earth. Allow yourself to notice how that energy feels throughout your entire body. You thank the tree for sharing its grounded energy, and it thanks you for noticing. Remember that you can come back to this tree anytime you wish.

Now take in a deep, energizing breath and return your awareness to the chair you are sitting in and the sounds in the room around you. Wiggle your fingers and toes. Move around a bit and stretch your body wherever it needs. Take in one more invigorating breath and open your eyes.

. . . .

Clearing Rain Meditation

The purpose of this meditation is to feel like you are washing away and clearing your energy field. Sometimes we feel drained or "off" after being around certain people or places. This meditation can be helpful in such cases.

I want you to utilize sound for this meditation to notice how it adds sensory focus and enhances the depth of the meditation. If you are doing this meditation from memory or having someone read it to you, first turn on some kind of rain noise. You may already have a sound machine or a CD or audio file with rain noise, or maybe it is actually raining where you are. If you do not have a rain sound readily available, here are three choices of websites/apps where you can listen to very nice nature and rain sounds for free:

> https://rain.today/
> http://www.noisli.com/
> http://mynoise.net/.

Many sensitive people find that sound generators with nature or other calming sounds are very helpful to aid work and study by drowning out less-wanted noises. These sounds can also be a great adjunct to deepen meditation as demonstrated below.

Begin by turning on a rain noise that you like. Sit and listen to it with your eyes closed for a few moments to make sure that it is at a perfect, soft volume so you can hear it well, but it will not interfere with listening to this meditation. Also make sure you really like the rain sound and that it naturally relaxes and calms you. So do that for a few moments ... listen to the rain sound and notice how it affects your breathing ... notice how it calms your thoughts ... notice how it seems to magically relax all your muscles. The sounds of nature can do that ... Take in a nice, slow, deep breath ... and then slowly, completely exhale ... and again ... breathing in ... and long, slow exhale.

Now tune in to your body ... Feel your clothing against your skin ... Feel your lungs expand as you breathe in and relax as you breathe out ... You may even be able to feel your heartbeat within your chest. Now expand your awareness outward. We all have a magnetic field. Our energy extends beyond our physical body ... Imagine that now. Your energetic field begins deep within your body and extends out past your internal organs through your skin ... outward ... extending outward around your body ... However far it seems to go is just fine.

Now tune back in to the sound of the rain. This is a very cleansing, clearing energetic rain that will rain down right into your energy field and into your body to loosen, clear, and release anything that is unneeded. It doesn't get you wet. It is made of the energy of rain. When you look up, you see this rain is coming from high, high up above the earth. Imagine this cleansing, energetic rain falling, falling, falling down … every drop meets your energy and renews it. All the thousands of drops pleasantly, gently rain down … refreshing you, clearing and renewing your energy … The rain travels through your energy field into your body, clearing any tension, any unneeded energy.

As this clearing rain continues to fall and refresh your energy and your body, you notice that it continues to fall straight down into the earth taking any unwanted energy to be recycled into pure, neutral energy … The rain falls from up high, high in the atmosphere, meeting your energetic field, raining down through it, through your body, and down, down, deep into the earth … down to the very core of the earth where it takes the unneeded energies to be transformed.

Spend the next few moments just listening to the sound of this rain … just listen to the sound … feel it clear and transform everything that is unneeded … leaving you refreshed … renewed … invigorated … because you now can clearly feel the energizing white light at your core that shines brightly. The rain has washed away all debris that was clouding the light … Now the light glows brightly, and you can feel it radiating out, giving you a steady stream of vitality.

Thank the rain for its purifying energy and know that you can quickly do this meditation again any and every time you hear the sound of rain. Now turn your attention back to the chair you are sitting in and the room you are in. Take in a very energizing breath and exhale. Wiggle your toes and fingers. Stretch a bit and open your eyes.

. . . .

Calming Aromatherapy Meditation

Sometimes when we are stressed, it can feel very frustrating to try to relax because our breathing gets stuck in tense, shallow mode. In this meditation we are going to use a natural scent (nothing synthetic please) to make it easy to relax right away.

Inhaling a scent you like will automatically deepen and slow your breathing, no effort required. So before we begin this guided meditation, please go get an aroma to inhale. Examples are a bottle of essential oil of lavender or sandalwood, a piece of orange, or a freshly cut aromatic flower or herb. Any natural scent that you really like will work.

For the meditation below, we are going to use a bottle of lavender essential oil, but you can modify it to use any scent you have or prefer.

Begin by sitting comfortably with your back supported. Take the bottle of essential oil in your hand. Close your eyes and first just notice how that item feels in your hand. How heavy is it? Can you feel the smooth glass? Roll it easily in your hands. Now think about how this lavender oil was made. Many, many lavender leaves and flowers were harvested. Where do you imagine the lavender flowers in your bottle were from?

Now take the cap off your bottle and bring it right up close to your nose to inhale. Deeply inhale the fresh scent, then slowly exhale. Notice how your breath in was slower and deeper simply by inhaling this scent. So let's focus on that this time, gently breathing in the scent as deeply as you can ... then pause for a moment ... and exhale slowly. And this time, I want you to notice how long the scent seems to linger in your nose before you fully exhale. Breathing in ... how long does the scent linger? And exhale.

Take a moment now and imagine a beautiful place in France where there is a huge field of lavender plants. You've never seen so many thousands of flowers all in one place. The landscape is also beautiful with rolling hills and trees off in the distance. Your eyes are elated with all the rich colors in the scene. The sky is deep blue with perfect sunshine and puffy white clouds. The lavender field is gorgeous shades of purple and green. Imagine you are up on a little hill with a perfect view of the lavender field. The fresh aroma from this many flowers fills the air all around. Inhale your scent again and imagine being right there breathing in the fresh scent of the lavender field. And take in one more energizing, deep breath. Know that you can return to this lovely place anytime you need a calming break.

Now return your attention to the room you are in. Open your eyes, and put the cap back on your bottle. Stretch your body wherever it feels it needs, and notice for a moment how much calmer your body feels and how much more deeply you can breathe now than when we started. Breathe in one more deep, invigorating breath and fully exhale.

. . . .

Connecting with Flower Essences Meditation

The purpose of this meditation is to prepare your mind and body for taking flower essences. It isn't necessary at all to do this meditation for the flower essences to work. You'll see though that this guided meditation is helpful to prepare your physical body and mind to fully accept and use the energies that the flower essences offer.

Sit comfortably, with your back supported and your feet flat on the floor. Close your eyes and take in a slow, relaxing breath and exhale. Shift around a bit or adjust your clothing if needed so you feel very comfortable. Take in another relaxing breath ... and exhale.

Begin with your awareness at the top of your head. Allow a heavy relaxation to flow down from the top of your head, slowly down, down. Down past your eyes so the muscles around your eyes relax and your eyes feel heavy ... The relaxation flows down your cheeks and down to your jaw, so that your jaw feels relaxed and heavy, falling open just a bit so your lips part slightly ... The relaxation continues to flow down your neck and throat ... down into your shoulders and down your arms. Your arms feel very heavy which pulls down your shoulders, relaxing them even more. The relaxing sensation flows down your chest and back ... down your belly and down into your legs, so that your legs feel very, very warm and heavy ... flowing all the way down your legs ... until the relaxation spills out the bottom of your feet ... Your entire body feels calm ... it is easy to breathe in slowly and deeply ... and exhale.

Now imagine that you are in a place where there are many, many flowering plants. This may be a garden of some kind or it may be a natural place with wildflowers. Whatever occurs to you is just right, but you do notice that all of your favorite flowers are there as well as some flowers you have never seen before. Take a moment and really look around the scene. The flowers are so many different colors and sizes. Notice what else is around. Trees, birds, maybe there is a pond or a stream. Look up in the sky and notice where the sun is and what kind of clouds are in the sky today. Take in all the sights and colors of this beautiful place.

Now breathe in deeply and notice how lovely the air smells from the gentle scents of the blossoms. There also is the fresh scent from the trees ...

Listen to the sounds you hear in this place. There are several different kinds of birds fluttering about. Hear their different sounds. You may hear the wind rustle the leaves of the trees and the sounds of squirrels and other animals scurrying about. Notice what else you hear in this place.

Now feel free to touch the bark of one of the trees and notice its roughness. Then bend down and lightly touch the petals of one of the flowers and notice how soft it is ... Feel the warmth of the sun and the gentle breeze on your skin ... Take in all the sights, sounds, and experiences of this place.

Now it suddenly occurs to you that all these plants have roots that grow underground, so that below the surface of the dirt is just as busy as it is above. You can feel all the various roots that grow in all different sizes and ways down into the soil and dirt, pulling up nutrients and water for the plants. As you stand amidst the flowers, you imagine that you also have roots growing from the bottom of your feet that intermingle with the roots of the plants so that you begin to really feel the energy of each plant as that energy rises up through your roots and into your body ... And that is how you begin to notice that each flower has its own ener-

gy and its own personality. Each plant has its own healing energy that it wants to share with you.

And it occurs to you how you never noticed before, but now you know that each and every flower you pass wherever you are has healing energy to help all of us humans who share the earth with them ... You take in a deep breath and feel all of this healing energy from nature enter your body ... allowing you stand up straighter ... feel stronger ... and more alive.

Take a look around again that this beautiful garden of flowers and know that you can return to this place as often as you want ... Take in an energizing breath ... and exhale. Bring your attention back to the chair you are sitting in and the sounds of the room around you. Wiggle your fingers and toes and stretch your body a bit ... When you are ready, open your eyes.

Resources/Bibliography

Books

Intuition & Empathic Development

Bodine, Echo. *A Still, Small Voice: A Psychic's Guide to Awakening Intuition*. Novato, CA: New World Library, 2001.

Brandon, Diane. *Intuition for Beginners: Easy Ways to Awaken Your Natural Abilities*. Woodbury, MN: Llewellyn, 2013.

Dale, Cyndi. *The Spiritual Power of Empathy: Develop Your Intuitive Gifts for Compassionate Connection*. Woodbury, MN: Llewellyn, 2014.

Dillard, Sherrie. *Discover Your Psychic Type: Developing and Using Your Natural Intuition*. Woodbury, MN: Llewellyn, 2008.

Peirce, Penney. *The Intuitive Way: The Definitive Guide to Increasing Your Awareness*. New York: Atria Books/Beyond Words, 2009.

Sanders, Pete A. *You Are Psychic!: The Free Soul Method*. New York: Ballantine, 1990.

EFT

Hass, Rue. *EFT for the Highly Sensitive Temperament*. Fulton, CA: Energy Psychology Press, 2009.

Solomon, Kathilyn. *Tapping Into Wellness: Using EFT to Clear Emotional & Physical Pain & Illness*. Woodbury, MN: Llewellyn, 2015.

Flower Essence Therapy

Kaminski, Patricia, and Richard Katz. *Flower Essence Repertory: A Comprehensive Guide to North American and English Flower Essences for Emotional and Spiritual Well-Being.* Nevada City, CA: Flower Essence Society, 1994.

Vennells, David. *Bach Flower Remedies for Beginners: 38 Essences that Heal from Deep Within.* Woodbury, MN: Llewellyn, 2001.

Herbalism/Spirit of Plants

Silvana, Laura. *Plant Spirit Journey: Discover the Healing Energies of the Natural World.* Woodbury, MN: Llewellyn, 2009.

Wood, Matthew. *The Book of Herbal Wisdom: Using Plants as Medicines.* Berkeley, CA: North Atlantic Books, 1997.

Mindfulness & Meditation

Clement, Stephanie. *Meditation for Beginners: Techniques for Awareness, Mindfulness & Relaxation.* Woodbury, MN: Llewellyn, 2002.

Jackson Brown, Freddy. *Get the Life You Want: Finding Meaning and Purpose through Acceptance and Commitment Therapy.* London, England: Watkins, 2013.

Nhat Hanh, Thich. *You Are Here: Discovering the Magic of the Present Moment.* Boston, MA: Shambhala, 2010.

Sciandra, Kate. *The Mindfulness Habit: Six Weeks to Creating the Habit of Being Present.* Woodbury, MN: Llewellyn, 2015.

Williams, Mark, John Teasdale, Zindel Segal, and Jon Kabat-Zinn. *The Mindful Way Through Depression: Freeing Yourself from Chronic Unhappiness.* New York: Guilford, 2007.

Our Energetic Existence

Becker, Robert, and Gary Selden. *The Body Electric: Electromagnetism and the Foundation of Life.* New York: William Morrow, 1998.

Emoto, Masaru. *The Hidden Messages in Water.* New York: Atria Books, 2005.

Pert, Candace, and Nancy Marriott. *Everything You Need to Know to Feel Go(o)d.* Carlsbad, CA: Hay House, 2007.

Websites

Sensitivity Websites & Blogs

Dr. Kyra's website, podcast, and videos:
   http://www.drkyra.com

Gentle Living Blog: http://gentlelivingonline.com

Elaine Aron's website: http://hsperson.com

A Highly Sensitive Person's Life Blog & Podcast:
   http://highlysensitiveperson.net

Sensitive Leadership: Changing the Way We Use Sensitivity:
   http://www.sensitiveleadership.com

Sensitive New World Blog: https://sensitivenewworld.wordpress.com

Sound Generators

Rain Today: https://rain.today

Noisli: http://www.noisli.com

My Noise: http://mynoise.net

Other Websites

EFT for Your Inner Child: http://eftforyourinnerchild.com

The Pocket Mindfulness Blog: http://www.pocketmindfulness.com

Index

J
journal, 2, 86, 139

K
Kabat-Zinn, Jon, 116
Keep Track of Negative Thoughts exercise, 112, 119
kinesiology, 132

L
lavender, 82, 158, 161, 174
Lesotho, 124
less-sensitive people, 12, 17, 19–21, 27, 39, 42, 49, 53, 67, 142, 144

M
magnetic resonance imaging, 21
manspreaders, 143
meditation, 44–46, 49, 55, 78, 100, 107–109, 114–116, 120, 121, 137–139, 155, 156, 159, 169, 171–175
Mindful Eating exercise, 116
Mindful Listening exercise, 117
Mindful Mundane Chore exercise, 118
Mindful Object Acknowledgement exercise, 118
Mindful Olfactory Sense exercise, 118
Mindful Shower exercise, 119
Mindful Walking exercise, 117
mindfulness, 78, 100, 107, 108, 111, 115–117, 119–121, 136
Mindfulness Based Stress Reduction, 116
Mister Rogers' Neighborhood, 109
mother earth, 78
muscle testing, 132–135, 137
Muscle Testing "Yes–No" Intuition Exercise, 133

N

Never-ending Sensitivity Syndrome (NESS), 91, 93, 94, 99, 103

P

perceptive, 6, 7, 11, 12, 15–21, 24, 39, 48, 65, 102, 115, 123, 146

Pert, Candace, 28–30, 33

pets, 36, 37, 127

physical stimuli, 12

plants, 7, 38, 43, 61, 75–88, 100, 118, 136, 137, 149, 155–157, 159–166, 174–177

positive deconstruction, 101, 102, 132

protection, 59, 60, 82, 160–162, 164–166

psychic, 48–50, 59, 60, 123, 124, 136, 158, 159, 164–166

Q

quantum components of sensitivity, 24, 25, 29, 31–33, 36, 37, 39, 43, 47–50, 54, 66, 72, 75, 76, 82–84, 87, 88, 102, 123, 124, 130

R

radiation, 27, 159, 160

rain, 171–173

Raisin Exercise, 116, 117

Reiki, 79, 100

resonance of energy, 59

Rogers, Fred, 109, 110

S

Sanders, Pete, 50, 179

Selwood, Ursula, 88, 165

Sheehan, Molly, 61, 137, 140

sensory processing sensitivity, 21, 22

Sensitivity Free Association Writing Exercise, 16

To Write to the Author

If you wish to contact the author or would like more information about this book, please write to the author in care of Llewellyn Worldwide Ltd. and we will forward your request. Both the author and publisher appreciate hearing from you and learning of your enjoyment of this book and how it has helped you. Llewellyn Worldwide Ltd. cannot guarantee that every letter written to the author can be answered, but all will be forwarded. Please write to:

Kyra Mesich, PsyD
℅ Llewellyn Worldwide
2143 Wooddale Drive
Woodbury, MN 55125-2989
Please enclose a self-addressed stamped envelope for reply,
or $1.00 to cover costs. If outside the USA, enclose
an international postal reply coupon.

Many of Llewellyn's authors have websites with
additional information and resources. For more information,
please visit our website at http://www.llewellyn.com.

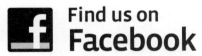
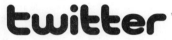

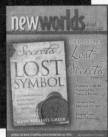

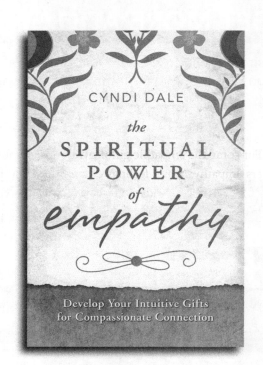

The Spiritual Power of Empathy
Develop Your Intuitive Gifts for Compassionate Connection
Cyndi Dale

For some the empathic gift provides insight and inspiration, but for others empathy creates feelings of confusion and panic. *The Spiritual Power of Empathy* is a hands-on training course for empaths, showing you how to comfortably use this often-unrecognized ability for better relationships, career advancement, raising children, and healing the self and others.

Join popular author Cyndi Dale as she shares ways to develop the six empathic types, techniques for screening and filtering information, and tips for opening up to a new world of deeper connections with the loved ones in your life. Also includes important information for dealing with the difficulties empaths often face, such as being overwhelmed in a crowd.

978-0-7387-3799-7, 264 pp., 6 x 9   **$16.99**

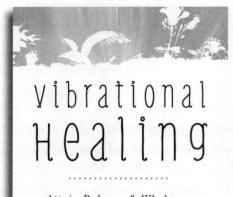

vibrational
Healing

· · · · · · · · · · · · · · · · · · · ·

Attain Balance & Wholeness

Understand Your Energetic Type

JAYA JAYA MYRA

Vibrational Healing
Attain Balance & Wholeness
Understand Your Energetic Type
JAYA JAYA MYRA

Explore the dynamic relationship between energy and health, and determine which vibrational healing techniques will work best for you. With simple questions designed to reveal your energy type, physical-body type, temperament, and purpose, *Vibrational Healing* is the perfect guide to creating a more balanced, vibrant, and healthy life.

Empowering and user-friendly, this remarkable book provides practical instructions for working with a variety of healing modalities, including:

Visualization • mantra • color • sound • light • aromatherapy • stones • water • intention • plants • meditation • minerals • herbs • and more

Join Jaya Jaya Myra as she shares the wealth of knowledge and insight she's gained from years of study with enlightened masters. Now is the time to customize a natural healing program just for you.

978-0-7387-4362-2, 240 pp., 5³⁄₁₆ x 8   **$15.99**

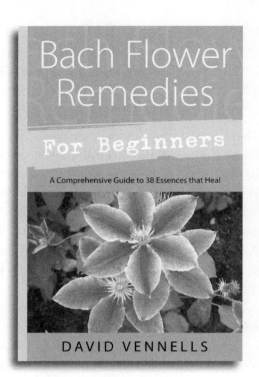

Bach Flower Remedies
For Beginners

A Comprehensive Guide to 38 Essences that Heal

DAVID VENNELLS

Bach Flower Remedies for Beginners
38 Essences that Heal from Deep Within
DAVID VENNELLS

The mind and body cannot be separated—what affects one will affect the other. The Bach Flower Remedies contain the subtle vibrational essences of flowers and trees. These remedies correct imbalances in the mental, emotional and spiritual bodies, promoting healing in the physical body.

Every day we are subjected to thousands of distractions, stressors, and pollutants. These myriad influences can wear down our natural defenses and cause frustration, tension, and even physical illness. The 38 Bach Flower Remedies are a safe and natural solution to the challenges of life in the 21st century. The remedies purify and balance the internal energy system, which in turn heals existing health problems—and can even help prevent future problems from manifesting!

Flower remedies are a safe and gentle form of alternative healing. They cannot harm—they only heal. In fact, they can even be given to children, animals, and plants.

978-0-7387-0047-2, 312 pp., 5³⁄₁₆ x 8   **$15.99**

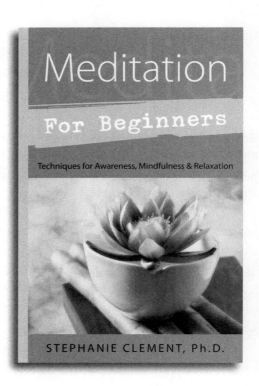

Meditation

For Beginners

Techniques for Awareness, Mindfulness & Relaxation

STEPHANIE CLEMENT, Ph.D.

Meditation for Beginners
Techniques for Awareness, Mindfulness & Relaxation
STEPHANIE CLEMENT, PhD

Break the barrier between your conscious and unconscious minds.

Perhaps the greatest boundary we set for ourselves is the one between the conscious and less conscious parts of our own minds. We all need a way to gain deeper understanding of what goes on inside our minds when we are awake, asleep, or just not paying attention. Meditation is one way to pay attention long enough to find out.

Meditation for Beginners offers a step-by-step approach to meditation, with exercises that introduce you to the rich possibilities of this age-old spiritual practice. Improve concentration, relax your body quickly and easily, work with your natural healing ability, and enhance performance in sports and other activities. Just a few minutes each day is all that's needed.

- Contains step-by-step meditation exercises
- Shows how to develop a consistent meditation effort in just a few minutes each day
- Explores many different ways to meditate, including kundalini yoga, walking meditation, dream meditation, tarot meditations, healing meditation.

978-0-7387-0203-2, 264 pp., 5³⁄₁₆ x 8   **$13.95**